T0195437

Office-Based Procedures: Part I

Editors

J. LANE WILSON
JONATHON FIRNHABER

PRIMARY CARE:
CLINICS IN OFFICE PRACTICE

www.primarycare.theclinics.com

Consulting Editor
JOEL J. HEIDELBAUGH

December 2021 • Volume 48 • Number 4

ELSEVIER

1600 John F. Kennedy Boulevard • Suite 1800 • Philadelphia, Pennsylvania, 19103-2899

http://www.theclinics.com

PRIMARYPRIMARY CARE: CLINICS IN OFFICE PRACTICE Volume 48, Number 4
December 2021 ISSN 0095-4543, ISBN-13: 978-0-323-80924-5

Editor:Editor: Katerina Heidhausen
Developmental Editor: Jessica Cañaberal

© 2021 Elsevier Inc. All rights reserved.

ThisThis periodical and the individual contributions contained in it are protected under copyright by Elsevier, and the following terms and conditions apply to their use:

Photocopying
Single photocopies of single articles may be made for personal use as allowed by national copyright laws. Permission of the Publisher and payment of a fee is required for all other photocopying, including multiple or systematic copying, copying for advertising or promotional purposes, resale, and all forms of document delivery. Special rates are available for educational institutions that wish to make photocopies for non-profit educational classroom use. For information on how to seek permission visit www.elsevier.com/permissions or call: (+44) 1865 843830 (UK)/(+1) 215 239 3804 (USA).

Derivative Works
Subscribers may reproduce tables of contents or prepare lists of articles including abstracts for internal circulation within their institutions. Permission of the Publisher is required for resale or distribution outside the institution. Permission of the Publisher is required for all other derivative works, including compilations and translations (please consult www.elsevier.com/permissions).

Electronic Storage or Usage
Permission of the Publisher is required to store or use electronically any material contained in this periodical, including any article or part of an article (please consult www.elsevier.com/permissions). Except as outlined above, no part of this publication may be reproduced, stored in a retrieval system or transmitted in any form or by any means, electronic, mechanical, photocopying, recording or otherwise, without prior written permission of the Publisher.

Notice
No responsibility is assumed by the Publisher for any injury and/or damage to persons or property as a matter of products liability, negligence or otherwise, or from any use or operation of any methods, products, instructions or ideas contained in the material herein. Because of rapid advances in the medical sciences, in particular, independent verification of diagnoses and drug dosages should be made.

Although all advertising material is expected to conform to ethical (medical) standards, inclusion in this publication does not constitute a guarantee or endorsement of the quality or value of such product or of the claims made of it by its manufacturer.

Primary Care: Clinics in Office Practice (ISSN: 0095-4543) is published quarterly by Elsevier Inc., 360 Park Avenue South, New York, NY 10010-1710. Months of issue are March, June, September, and December. Periodicals postage paid at New York, NY and additional mailing offices. Subscription prices are $261.00 per year (US individuals), $649.00 (US institutions), $100.00 (US students), $303.00 (Canadian individuals), $688.00 (Canadian institutions), $100.00 (Canadian students), $357.00 (international individuals), $688.00 (international institutions), and $175.00 (international students). Foreign air speed delivery is included in all *Clinics* subscription prices. All prices are subject to change without notice. POSTMASTER: Send address changes to *Primary Care: Clinics in Office Practice*, Elsevier Periodicals Customer Service, 11830 Westline Industrial Drive, St. Louis, MO 63146. Customer Service Health Sciences Division, Subscription Customer Service, 3251 Riverport Lane, Maryland Heights, MO 63043. **Customer Service: 1-800-654-2452 (U.S. and Canada); 314-447-8871 (outside U.S. and Canada). Fax: 314-447-8029. E-mail: journalscustomerservice-usa@elsevier.com (for print support); journalsonlinesupport-usa@elsevier.com (for online support).**

Reprints. For copies of 100 or more, of articles in this publication, please contact the Commercial Reprints Department, Elsevier Inc., 360 Park Avenue South, New York, NY 10010-1710. Tel. 212-633-3874; Fax: 212-633-3820; E-mail: reprints@elsevier.com.

Primary Care: Clinics in Office Practice is covered in *MEDLINE/PubMed (Index Medicus)* and *EMBASE/ Excerpta Medica, Current Contents/Clinical Medicine, and ISI/BIOMED.*

Contributors

CONSULTING EDITOR

JOEL J. HEIDELBAUGH, MD, FAAFP, FACG
Clinical Professor, Departments of Family Medicine and Urology, Director of Medical
Student Education and Clerkship Director, Department of Family Medicine, University of
Michigan Medical School, Ann Arbor, Michigan; Ypsilanti Health Center, Ypsilanti, Michigan

EDITORS

J. LANE WILSON, MD
Assistant Professor of Family Medicine, Brody School of Medicine, East Carolina
University, ECU Family Medicine Center, Greenville, North Carolina

JONATHON FIRNHABER, MD, MAEd, MBA
Professor of Family Medicine, Brody School of Medicine, East Carolina University, ECU
Family Medicine Center, Greenville, North Carolina

AUTHORS

LOREN COLSON, DO
Faculty, Family Medicine Residency of Idaho, Boise, Idaho; Clinical Instructor, University
of Washington, Department of Family Medicine

JONATHON FIRNHABER, MD, MAEd, MBA
Professor of Family Medicine, Brody School of Medicine, East Carolina University, ECU
Family Medicine Center, Greenville, North Carolina

KRYSTAL FOSTER, MD
Assistant Professor of Clinical Family and Community Medicine, Department of Family and
Community Medicine, University of Missouri, Columbia, Missouri

BERNADATTE G. GILBERT, MD
Assistant Professor/Staff Physician, Department of Family and Community Medicine,
Penn State Health Milton S. Hershey Medical Center, Penn State College of Medicine,
Hershey, Pennsylvania; Penn State Health Medical Group, Harrisburg, Pennsylvania

MADELINE HAAS, MD
Assistant Professor, Department of Family and Community Medicine, Albany Medical
College, Albany, New York

FADI HANNA, MD
Department of Family and Community Medicine, Wake Forest School of Medicine,
Winston-Salem, North Carolina

VASUDHA JAIN, MD
MUSC Affiliate Assistant Professor, Tidelands Health Family Medicine Residency
Program, Myrtle Beach, South Carolina

NATALIE LONG, MD
Assistant Professor of Clinical Family and Community Medicine, Department of Family and Community Medicine, University of Missouri, Columbia, Missouri

STEPHANIE LONG, MD, FAAFP
Community Faculty, Clinical Instructor, Department of Family Medicine, University of Washington, Seattle, Washington; Family Medicine Residency of Idaho, Boise, Idaho

ANDREW LUTZKANIN, MD, FAAFP
Assistant Professor, Department of Family and Community Medicine, Penn State Health Hershey Medical Center, Hershey, Pennsylvania

MICHAEL MALONE, MD, DIO
Program Director, Tidelands Health Family Medicine Residency Program, Myrtle Beach, South Carolina

LAQUITA MORRIS, MD
Assistant Professor of Clinical Family and Community, Department of Family and Community Medicine, University of Missouri, Columbia, Columbia, Missouri

KIRAN MULLUR, MD
Department of Family and Community Medicine, Wake Forest School of Medicine, Winston-Salem, North Carolina

SARAH INÉS RAMÍREZ, MD, FAAFP
Assistant Professor, Department of Family and Community Medicine, Penn State Health Hershey Medical Center, Hershey, Pennsylvania

BRIAN RAYALA, MD
Professor, Department of Family Medicine, The University of North Carolina at Chapel Hill, Chapel Hill, North Carolina

ANNIE RUTTER, MD, MS, FAAFP
Associate Professor and Academic Vice Chair, Department of Family and Community Medicine, Albany Medical College, Albany, New York

MELANIE H. SANDERS, MD
Clinical Assistant Professor, Department of Family Medicine, Brody School of Medicine, East Carolina University, Greenville, North Carolina

HEATH C. THORNTON, MD, CAQSM
Associate Professor, Department of Family and Community Medicine, Wake Forest School of Medicine, Winston-Salem, North Carolina

BRIDGID HAST WILSON, MD, PhD
Clinical Assistant Professor of Family Medicine, Brody School of Medicine, East Carolina University, Greenville, North Carolina

J. LANE WILSON, MD
Assistant Professor of Family Medicine, Brody School of Medicine, East Carolina University, ECU Family Medicine Center, Greenville, North Carolina

MATTHEW ZEITLER, MD
Clinical Assistant Professor, Department of Family Medicine, The University of North Carolina at Chapel Hill, Chapel Hill, North Carolina

Contents

Intrauterine devices (IUDs) are safe, highly effective, reversible contraception and come in 2 varieties in the United States: nonhormonal (copper) or levonorgestrel hormonal (LNG) IUDs. There are few absolute contraindications, making them appropriate birth control for most patients. Patients are more likely to select an IUD when counseled about IUD removal and factors that are important to them. IUD insertion and removal are uncomplicated office procedures that can be offered by primary care providers.

Nexplanon is the only contraceptive implant currently available in the United States. It exerts its contraceptive effects primarily by suppressing ovulation. The Nexplanon is the most effective method of long-acting reversible contraception. The implant should be removed by the end of the third year of use. Persons will experience a rapid return to fertility once the implant is removed. All health care providers must be trained on Nexplanon before performing insertions or removals of the implant. A Nexplanon can be inserted and/or removed as an office-based procedure. The most common adverse reaction is change in menstrual bleeding patterns.

Abnormal uterine bleeding is a frequent medical concern for premenopausal and postmenopausal patients. Endometrial biopsy is a safe, cost-effective option offered in the office setting. Although endometrial biopsy may result in insufficient tissue or false-negative results, data suggest that endometrial biopsy is 90% sensitive for endometrial cancer and 82% sensitive for atypical hyperplasia, with specificity of 100% for postmenopausal patients and similar results in premenopausal patients. Topical cervical analgesia and oral nonsteroidal anti-inflammatory drugs decrease a patient's discomfort during endometrial biopsy. Aftercare instructions and how patients want to receive results should be reviewed in advance of performing the endometrial biopsy.

While Bartholin gland abscesses are less commonly seen outpatient pathology, prompt diagnosis and treatment are essential to preventing serious complications such as sepsis and rectovaginal fistula. Owing to an unacceptably high recurrence rate, simple incision and drainage is insufficient for primary treatment; preferably, placement of a Word catheter or Jacobi ring device to reepithelize the duct may be done under local anesthesia in an outpatient clinic. Destruction of the gland through silver nitrate application or alcohol sclerotherapy is an alternative. Marsupialization is often reserved for recurrent cases, although can be offered as primary management in some situations.

Declining cervical cancer rates in the United States highlights the value of prevention and early detection of premalignant cervical disease afforded by the human papillomavirus vaccine and Pap smear. The availability of in-office loop electrosurgical excision procedure affords clinicians with a cost-effective and preferred tool for the excision of high-grade lesions of the cervix with minimal risk for severe adverse outcomes. The most recent American Society for Colposcopy and Cervical Pathology guidelines recommend a risk-based approach for the detection, treatment, and surveillance of cervical disease and specifically focus on the risk of developing cervical intraepithelial neoplasia 3 or worse histology.

Neonatal circumcision is one of the most common elective surgical procedures in the United States and globally. This procedure, to remove part of the penile prepuce or foreskin, is done for a variety of personal, social, and medical reasons. There are several proposed benefits, risks, and ethical considerations to discuss with parents before the procedure. Three equally safe and effective methods are used for circumcision, and each uses unique equipment: the Gomco clamp, the Mogen clamp, and the Plastibell device. Choice of technique should be guided by operator training and comfort.

Vasectomy is a safe, effective, and practical option for permanent contraception in men. Vasectomy is a surgical procedure used in men to disrupt and occlude the vas deferens, which delivers sperm from the testicles. By interrupting sperm transport, this procedure provides permanent sterilization. Vasectomies are typically done under local anesthesia in outpatient settings, and patients usually go home within an hour of the surgery. Surgical techniques used for vasectomy vary widely throughout the world, with limited evidence to guide the most effective approach. Current

Office-based laboratory and bedside diagnostic procedures can be a helpful tool when assessing patients in the ambulatory setting. Diagnostic tests using a microscope (including assessment of vaginal discharge, urinary sediment, or skin scraping) or a diagnostic ultraviolet (UV) light (when evaluating the cornea or skin) can add valuable information to aid in proper diagnosis. This chapter will review necessary materials, technique, and interpretation for these often simple and inexpensive evaluations.

Pediatric patients are frequently evaluated in primary care clinics. Thus, there exists a need to understand common pediatric problems and to acquire a degree of familiarity with pediatric procedures. This article will review techniques and the current evidence for frequently performed pediatric procedures, including umbilical granuloma chemocautery, frenotomy, suture ligation of type B postaxial polydactyly, reduction of nursemaid's elbow, hair tourniquet removal, and tympanometry.

PRIMARY CARE:
CLINICS IN OFFICE PRACTICE

SERIES OF RELATED INTEREST

Medical Clinics (http://www.medical.theclinics.com)
Physician Assistant Clinics (https://www.physicianassistant.theclinics.com)

THE CLINICS ARE AVAILABLE ONLINE!
Access your subscription at:
www.theclinics.com

Foreword

"Oh, You Can Do That?"

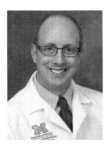

Joel J. Heidelbaugh, MD, FAAFP, FACG
Consulting Editor

I went to medical school to be a surgeon. At least, that's what I thought I wanted to become because I loved the prospect of doing procedures. I had no real knowledge of primary care, what it encompassed, and what a career in primary care could provide for my patients. Just last week one of my students said to me, *"I thought all you did in primary care was physicals and refer patients to specialists."* Yes, we've all heard this inaccurate stigma before, and we've all tried to successfully break it down. While this is important to counter and clarify in medical education, it is perhaps equally or more important that we educate our patients that we can provide a wide palette of procedural care at the same level as our specialty colleagues. In a single day of patient care, I was approached by patients who wanted a referral to a dermatologist to remove a nevus, a referral to a podiatrist to treat a wart, and a referral to an orthopedic surgeon for a steroid injection in their knee. Each patient was overwhelmingly surprised that I could provide each of these services in my own office, without a significant wait time for a referral, on the same day that they requested the procedure, and the procedure would be performed by someone they know and already trust. And each patient exclaimed, *"Oh, you can do that?"*

In my family medicine residency, I stumbled upon Pfenninger and Fowler's landmark book, *"Procedures for Primary Care,"* which is now in its third edition. I was blown away at the prospect of how one could incorporate so many types of office-based procedures into daily practice. Not every primary care physician performs every procedure; not every specialist within a particular field practices every element of that field. Office-based procedures greatly add to the diversity of what clinicians can offer within their practices and can improve practice margins through additional revenue. Procedures can also help to define a niche within one's practice, including women's health, dermatology, and sports medicine; the list seems nearly endless.

As Drs Wilson and Firnhaber state in their preface, we should embrace the idea of including procedures in our daily practices and learning new skills over time.

Prim Care Clin Office Pract 48 (2021) xi–xii
https://doi.org/10.1016/j.pop.2021.07.012
0095-4543/21/© 2021 Published by Elsevier Inc.

Continuing medical education, additional training, and on-the-job mentorship have afforded many primary care physicians the opportunity to learn procedures postresidency and midcareer. Incorporating procedures into daily practice enhances our job satisfaction, and more importantly, shows our patients that we can provide a high degree of comprehensive care within the scope of our practices.

I would like to thank our expert guest editors and authors for their commitment to this, the first of 2 issues on office-based procedures in our *Primary Care: Clinics in Office Practice* series for primary care clinicians. These articles provide current and evidence-based approaches to common procedures well suited for primary care clinicians to be used readily in practice. If you already do some of these procedures, then you can augment your knowledge with new evidence and improve your skills. If you don't already do some of these procedures, then consider taking a course or learning from a colleague how to become proficient and credentialed, then expand the services you provide and your joy of the practice of primary care medicine.

Joel J. Heidelbaugh, MD, FAAFP, FACG
Departments of Family Medicine and Urology
University of Michigan Medical School
Ann Arbor, MI, USA

Ypsilanti Health Center
200 Arnet Suite 200
Ypsilanti, MI 48198, USA

E-mail address:
jheidel@umich.edu

Preface

Think of Yourself as a Comprehensivist

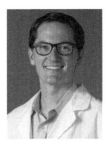 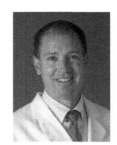

J. Lane Wilson, MD   Jonathon Firnhaber, MD, MAEd, MBA
Editors

What exactly is it that makes office-based procedures so much fun? There's got to be something, because as residency faculty, procedures training is one of the most common aspects of our program that applicants ask about. Residency applicants don't yet realize that procedures notes are quicker to write than typical clinic notes. They have not done enough procedures to appreciate the satisfaction that comes from performing an entire vasectomy through a tiny tear in the scrotum, or from reducing a Nursemaid elbow using just your hands. And they certainly haven't experienced flow—that psychological state also known as being "in the zone"—that is so difficult to achieve in other areas of practice but readily accompanies the hands-on action of procedural care. Maybe they already recognize the difference between a generalist and a "comprehensivist"—which is a term we've just made up. We are quite certain our patients appreciate that difference because they tell us all the time. And there are data to support the idea that physicians who perform office-based procedures have higher overall satisfaction with their practice.[1,2]

Most likely, you're reading this issue of *Primary Care: Clinics in Office Practice* because you've decided you'd like to *do more procedures*. The question is: which ones? That question has been debated for decades, by all sorts of well-intentioned and intelligent academic physicians, but there's still no consensus on which procedures *all* primary care physicians should be able to perform.[3,4] The Accreditation Council for Graduate Medical Education, while decidedly nonspecific, offers guidance that makes sense not just for residency programs but also for clinicians in the community: know how to perform the procedures that are most pertinent for your clinical setting and patient population. If you don't routinely see women of childbearing age, it's not critical for you to learn to place IUDs or contraceptive implants—and you can make the same argument for each of the procedures outlined in this issue or in its companion issue. But without question, we have covered at least one procedure that is both pertinent to your patient population and is not something you already do. Start there. Take advantage of the opportunity to take your fingers off a keyboard and put them on a patient. Reexperience that satisfaction of offering your patients truly comprehensive care and get reacquainted with saying, "I can take care of that for you." And start thinking of yourself as a comprehensivist.

J. Lane Wilson, MD
Brody School of Medicine
East Carolina University
ECU Family Medicine Center
101 Heart Drive
Greenville, NC 27834, USA

Jonathon Firnhaber, MD, MAEd, MBA
Brody School of Medicine
East Carolina University
ECU Family Medicine Center
101 Heart Drive
Greenville, NC 27834, USA

E-mail addresses:
wilsonjo@ecu.edu (J.L. Wilson)
firnhaberj@ecu.edu (J. Firnhaber)

REFERENCES

1. Weidner AKH, Phillips RL Jr, Fang B, et al. Burnout and scope of practice in new family physicians. Ann Fam Med 2018;16(3):200–5 [published correction appears in Ann Fam Med 2018;16(4):289].
2. Rivet C, Ryan B, Stewart M. Hands on: is there an association between doing procedures and job satisfaction? Can Fam Physician 2007;53(1):93, 93:e.1-5, 92.
3. Kelly BF, Sicilia JM, Forman S, et al. Advanced procedural training in family medicine: a group consensus statement. Fam Med 2009;41(6):398–404.
4. Nothnagle M, Sicilia JM, Forman S, et al. Required procedural training in family medicine residency: a consensus statement. Fam Med 2008;40(4):248–52.

Intrauterine Device Insertion and Removal

Stephanie Long, MD[a,b], Loren Colson, DO[a,b],*

KEYWORDS

- Intrauterine • Device • Levonorgestrel • LNG • Copper • IUD • Contraception
- LARC

KEY POINTS

- Intrauterine devices (IUDs) have been used for contraception for more than a century; however, they have had a significant decline in use in the 1970s followed by a re-emergence in the 2000s.
- There currently are 1 copper IUD and 4 levonorgestrel IUDs approved by the Food and Drug Administration (FDA), with considerable data supporting their safety and efficacy.
- There are few patients who are not appropriate candidates for 1 or all FDA-approved IUDs in the United States.
- Patient-centered counseling regarding method side effects and removal process is important to method uptake.
- Insertion and removal of IUDs are safe and simple office procedures.

INTRODUCTION

The purpose of this procedural guide is to provide guidance on patient-centered counseling, insertion, and removal for intrauterine devices (IUDs).

HISTORY/BACKGROUND

Although there are reports of IUDs being used for contraception dating back to the early 1900s, the first T-shaped device was designed in 1969 by Dr Howard Tatum. Dr Tatum created a simple plastic T, which was well tolerated but had a pregnancy rate of 18%. Around the same time, Dr Jaime Zipper had discovered that putting a copper wire in the uterus of a rabbit prevented pregnancy. Dr Tatum used this finding and, with the addition of copper wire in his T-shaped device, the pregnancy rate on the IUD decreased from 18% to approximately 1%.[1–4]

[a] Family Medicine Residency of Idaho, 777 North Raymond Street, Boise, ID 83704, USA;
[b] University of Washington, Department of Family Medicine, Seattle, WA, USA
* Corresponding author.
E-mail address: Loren.colson@fmridaho.org

Prim Care Clin Office Pract 48 (2021) 531–544
https://doi.org/10.1016/j.pop.2021.07.001
0095-4543/21/© 2021 Elsevier Inc. All rights reserved.
primarycare.theclinics.com

In 1970, Dr Antonio Scommegna devised a T-shaped device that contained a semipermeable progesterone capsule. It was approved by the Food and Drug Administration (FDA) for use for 1 year and was on the market until the early 2000s.[2,3]

In 1971, the A.H. Robins Company released an IUD known as the Dalkon Shield. It was marketed as highly effective with a very low adverse effect rate. Unfortunately, within a few years of being on the market there were thousands of reports of pelvic inflammatory disease, infertility, midtrimester abortion, and sepsis and 17 cases of death. This was thought to be caused by the braided removal string that allowed bacteria to travel up the string and into the uterus. Due to these complications and an overwhelming number of lawsuits, the Dalkon Shield was removed from the market in 1974, and A.H. Robins Company filed for bankruptcy soon thereafter. In the aftermath, there was a significant stigma in the United States around IUDs. All IUDs except for 1 progesterone-containing device were removed from the market, and IUD use significantly diminished for several years.[5,6]

After several years of decreased popularity, a new IUD appeared in 1988, the copper T 380A ParaGard. The FDA approved its use for 4 years, but as data accumulated, the effectiveness eventually was moved to up to 10 years. This was followed by a levonorgestrel (LNG)-releasing intrauterine system (Mirena) in 2001. This device and the ParaGard were shown to be highly effective and had a much better safety profile than the Dalkon Shield.[5,7,8]

In 2013 a LNG-containing IUD, Skyla by Bayer, was approved by the FDA. Skyla was designed to prevent pregnancy for 3 years and targeted to women who have not had children.[9]

Abbvie introduced the Liletta IUD, which gained FDA approval in 2015. It was marketed as a less expensive alternative to the Mirena IUD and contains the same amount of LNG.[10]

In 2016, Bayer announced that the FDA approved Kyleena, a progestin-containing intrauterine system, for the prevention of pregnancy for up to 5 years.[11]

These new IUDs have proved safe, effective, and low-risk forms of contraception that have seen increasing use over time. The proportion of women using long-acting, reversible contraceptive methods, such as the IUD, has risen from 2.0% in 2002 to 12% in 2014.[12]

FOOD AND DRUG ADMINISTRATION–APPROVED INTRAUTERINE DEVICES IN THE UNITED STATES

- ParaGard—https://www.paragard.com/
- Liletta—https://www.liletta.com/
- Mirena—https://www.mirena-us.com/
- Kyleena—https://www.kyleena-us.com/
- Skyla—https://www.skyla-us.com/

CHARACTERISTICS OF FOOD AND DRUG ADMINISTRATION–APPROVED INTRAUTERINE DEVICES IN THE UNITED STATES
Mechanisms of Action

Levonorgestrel intrauterine device
Hormonal IUDs release LNG, a progestin, causing cervical mucus to thicken so sperm cannot enter the fallopian tubes to reach ovum (**Table 1**). Changes in uterotubal fluid also impair sperm migration. Alteration of the endometrium prevents implantation of fertilized ovum. There also is some anovulatory effect.

Table 1
Comparative table of the Food and Drug Administration–approved intrauterine devices in the United States

| | Copper Intrauterine Device | Levonorgestrel Intrauterine Devices | | | |
	ParaGard	Liletta, 52 mg	Mirena, 52 mg	Kyleena, 19.5 mg	Skyla, 13.5 mg
Duration					
FDA approved	10 y	6 y	6 y	5 y	3 y
Evidence based (Wu)	12 y	7 y	7 y	N/A	N/A
Size (mm)	32 × 36	32 × 32	32 × 32	28 × 30	28 × 32
Effective for pregnancy prevention (after insertion)	Immediately	7 d; immediate if used for emergency contraception	7 d; immediate if used for emergency contraception	7 d	7 d
Consider for	Hormone-free option	Reduced cost option	Treatment of heavy menses (FDA approved)	Smaller IUD with long duration	Smallest IUD with lowest hormone dose

Data from Refs.[13–15]

Copper intrauterine device

ParaGard contains 176 mg of copper wire coiled along the vertical stem and a 68.7-mg collar on each side of the horizontal arm. Copper interferes with sperm transport and fertilization of an egg and may prevent implantation.

Efficacy

- All FDA-approved IUDs have a reported efficacy of greater than 99.[13]
- Emergency contraception
  - Copper IUDs can be inserted as emergency contraception for up to 5 days after unprotected intercourse.[16]
  - Data published in 2021 demonstrate comparable efficacy using the LNG, 52 mg, IUD (Mirena or Liletta) as emergency contraception for up to 5 days after unprotected intercourse. A backup contraceptive method is not needed for the 52-mg LNG IUDs when used as emergency contraceptive.[17] A backup method is recommended for a 52-mg LNG IUD start at any other time.

PREOPERATIVE/PREPROCEDURE PLANNING

- Contraceptive counseling and method selection
- Discussion of what to expect with the method
- Discussion of benefits/risks/alternatives and consent form
- Sexually transmitted infection (STI) testing if indicated by
  - Age-based risk with screening per US Preventive Services Task Force guidelines
  - Risk-based screening (Centers for Disease Control and Prevention [CDC], Sexually Transmitted Infections Treatment Guidelines https://www.cdc.gov/std/treatment)

o Patient request
- Determine that patient is not pregnant, including pregnancy test, as indicated (**Box 1**).

Counseling

Contraceptive counseling should include eliciting what matters to a patient about their birth control, screening for method safety, and preparation for method initiation (or insertion), and aftercare. Many online resources exist for patient counseling, including tools that compare methods as well as patient handouts. It also may be helpful to use demonstration kits, as shown below, for patients. Patients can touch the demonstration IUD as well as see where and how it is placed in the uterus.

Factors to Consider for Intrauterine Devices

- IUD removal
  - o Unlike other methods, where a patient may be able to self-discontinue their birth control, counseling about method removal is an important part of method selection.
  - o Patients should be reassured that their IUD can be removed at any time. Some are most comfortable doing this in the office, as discussed later. Others may prefer, or simply be reassured about the option, to self-remove their IUD.[20]
- Changes to menstrual cycle
  - o Copper IUD
    - Menstrual cycles are maintained with the copper IUD.
    - Menses may be heavier or longer with the copper IUD initially but may improve with continued use.[21]
    - If menstruation stops, patients should be evaluated for pregnancy and secondary amenorrhea.
  - o LNG IUDs
    - LNG may result in amenorrhea for some women and/or decrease in menstrual bleeding with some irregularity and/or spotting for many patients. There are more pronounced changes to menses with the 52-mg LNG devices compared with the 13.5 mg device.

Box 1
How can I be "reasonably certain" my patient is not pregnant?

According to the CDC, health care providers may use the following criteria to determine that a patient is reasonably not pregnant, with a 99% to 100% negative predictive value.

A patient is reasonably not pregnant if they have no symptoms or signs of pregnancy and meets any 1 of the following criteria:

- Is ≤ 7 days after the start of normal menses
- Has not had sexual intercourse since the start of last normal menses
- Has been correctly and consistently using a reliable method of contraception
- Is ≤ 7 days after spontaneous or induced abortion
- Is within 4 weeks postpartum
- Is fully or nearly fully breastfeeding (exclusively breastfeeding or the vast majority [$\geq 85\%$] of feeds are breastfeeds), amenorrheic, and less than 6 months postpartum.

Data from Refs.[18,19]

- Probability of amenorrhea after 1 year varies with the IUD[22]
  - Liletta: 1 in 5
  - Mirena: 1 in 5
  - Kyleena: 1 in 8
  - Skyla: 1 in 17
- Nulliparous patients and adolescents
  - IUD use in nulliparous and adolescent patients is supported by the American College of Obstetricians and Gynecologists (ACOG).[23]
- Ectopic pregnancy
  - Overall, rates of ectopic pregnancy are lower than in non-contracepting patients, given the efficacy of IUDs to prevent pregnancy.
  - If pregnancy occurs, however, it should be presumed to be ectopic until evaluation proves otherwise.
- Future fertility
  - Many patients ask about effects on future fertility. Once an IUD is removed, patients return to immediate fertility. Fertility changes, however, over time. Delaying the decision to seek pregnancy, and not the IUD, may change a patient's fertility when discontinuing an IUD.
- Cost
  - Although the overall costs of the IUD are lower than many methods over the life span of the IUD, the initial cost may be higher than those of other methods when the costs of the device and insertion are included. Cost varies based on insurance status and access to city, state, or other assistance programs.
- Other questions may arise when counseling patients. The following resources may be of benefit to providers and patients:
  - ACOG: https://www.acog.org/About-ACOG/ACOG-Departments/Long-Acting-Reversible-Contraception
  - Bedsider, an online birth control support network from Power to Decide
    - Bedsider Providers: https://providers.bedsider.org/
    - Bedsider IUDs: https://www.bedsider.org/methods/iud
  - Reproductive Health Access Project: https://www.reproductiveaccess.org/contraception/

DETERMINING ELIGIBILITY FOR THE INTRAUTERINE DEVICE

IUDs are appropriate for most patients. The CDC publishes and updates the US Medical Eligibility Criteria for Contraceptive Use, an evidence-based guideline for contraceptive method initiation and continuation based on medical conditions. It is available at   https://www.cdc.gov/reproductivehealth/contraception/pdf/summary-chart-us-medical-eligibilitycriteria_508tagged.pdf.

INFORMED CONSENT FOR INTRAUTERINE DEVICES

- Indications
  - Patients, nulliparous or parous, who want reliable or long-acting reversible contraception (LARC)
  - Specific for LNG IUDs
    - Women with heavy bleeding or painful menses
    - Menopausal women using hormone replacement therapy with intact uterus to prevent endometrial hyperplasia
    - Transgender patients on testosterone therapy who desire menstrual cessation and/or contraception

- ○ Specific for copper IUDs
  - ■ Desire LARC with continued menses
- • Contraindications
  - ○ Current or possible pregnancy
  - ○ Current sexually transmitted infection
  - ○ Recent pelvic inflammatory disease (within past 3 months)
  - ○ Uterus sounds to less than 6 cm or larger than 9 cm
- • Consider imaging and/or referral to a more experienced provider for insertion
  - ○ Uterine distortion or pathology
  - ○ Undiagnosed abnormal vaginal bleeding
  - ○ Current IUD in place or incomplete removal of prior IUD
  - ○ Allergy to a component of the device
    - ■ Hypersensitivity to a component
      - • The prescriber's information may help for specific components of the IUD selected for a patient (eg, Mirena contains LNG, silicone, polyethylene, silica, barium sulfate, or iron oxide).
    - ■ Metal allergies
      - • ParaGard contains copper
      - • Kyleena and Skyla contain a sterling silver ring
  - ○ Specific to LNG IUDs
    - ■ Active liver disease, as evidenced by jaundice, viral hepatitis, cirrhosis of the liver, or a liver tumor
    - ■ Confirmed or suspected progestin-sensitive cancer
  - ○ Specific to copper IUDs
    - ■ Significant anemia
    - ■ Wilson disease
    - ■ Copper allergy
- • Complications
  - ○ Infection: 0% to 2% risk[24]
    - ■ Slight increase risk of pelvic inflammatory disease within 20 days of insertion that increases with bacterial vaginitis, cervicitis, or contamination with insertion
  - ○ Perforation: 0.1% to 0.3% risk[25]
  - ○ Rare vasovagal reaction or fainting during insertion
  - ○ Embedded in uterus
  - ○ Expulsion
    - ■ Increased when not placed in fundus or placed immediately postpartum
  - ○ Difficult placement or failed insertion
  - ○ Pregnancy: 0.1% failure rate in first year[25]
  - ○ Ectopic pregnancy

EQUIPMENT
Intrauterine Device Insertion

- • Ring forceps (**Fig. 1**)
- • Single-tooth tenaculum
- • Scissors
  - ○ Angled-tip, long-handled scissors are recommended if available
- • Uterine sound, disposable plastic (as pictured) or metal reusable
- • Speculum
- • Large obstetrics swabs/scopettes or 4 × 4 gauze

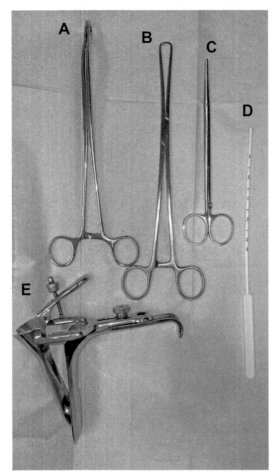

Fig. 1. Typical sterile procedure tray with necessary equipment for IUD insertion. A, Ring forceps; B, tenaculum; C, scissors; D, uterine sounds; and E, speculum.

- Gloves (sterile or nonsterile)
- Light source
- IUD selected by patient
  - Some providers keep the device sterile until they have successfully sounded the uterus to avoid wasting a device if it cannot be placed.

Intrauterine Device Removal

- Speculum
- Ring, forceps
- Gloves (sterile or nonsterile)
- Light source
- Large obstetric swabs/scopettes (optional)
- In cases of missing strings, the following instruments may be of benefit:
  - Cytobrush
  - IUD hook
  - Alligator forceps

　　　○ Serpentine grasper

Preparation and Patient Positioning

- Verify patient is reasonably not pregnant and appropriate for insertion that day.
- Consider if additional studies should be offered or collected during insertion:
  - Cervical cancer screening with pap smear
  - STI screening, if indicated
    - If results return positive, infection should be treated, per CDC guidelines (*Sexually Transmitted Infections Treatment Guidelines*).
- Ultrasound is not required but may be helpful, especially in cases of complications.
- Position patient in dorsal lithotomy position with use of foot or knee rests.
- Pain management
  - Oral agents—nonsteroidal anti-inflammatory drug (NSAID), such as ibuprofen, 800 mg, or Tylenol, 1000 mg
  - Cervical anesthesia
    - Paracervical block—an option for additional anesthesia, if needed, but not required routinely
      - If unable to tolerate procedure or per patient request, a paracervical block may be of benefit. More information on how to perform a paracervical block is available from the reproductive health organization, Ipas: https://www.ipas.org/wp-content/uploads/2020/06/PARABLK-E19.pdf.
    - Intracervical block—similar to a paracervical block but with intracervical application. This may be considered for patient comfort or with a difficult insertion.
  - Topical anesthetics—benzocaine spray (HurriCaine) or similar
- Cervical preparation
  - There is no evidence to support misoprostol use for routine IUD insertion; evidence suggests increased patient side effects without increasing the ease of insertion.[24]
  - If a failed first insertion and reattempt is desired, misoprostol may be considered.
- Cervical cleansing is recommended by manufacturers; however, there is little evidence to support that this reduces risk of intrauterine infection. If the decision to use an antiseptic is made, chlorhexidine is preferred over povidone-iodine.[26–28]
- No-touch technique
  - Some providers prefer to perform IUD insertions with sterile gloves. The use of sterile equipment and sterile gloves does not exclude contamination and it is common to employ a no-touch technique, meaning that the provider does not touch any sterile equipment that enters the uterus.[29]
  - Many large organizations have incorporated the no-touch technique in their IUD trainings,[30,31] and the benefit of no touch technique, even in aseptic settings, has been demonstrated.[32]

PROCEDURAL APPROACH
Intrauterine Device Insertion

1. Perform bimanual examination to determine uterine size and position.
2. Insert speculum into the vagina using a lubricant for patient comfort until cervix is visualized.
3. Maintain sterile no-touch technique.
4. Optionally, apply single-tooth tenaculum to cervix.

    a. Anterior position is most common.

    b. Posterior position may aid insertion in a retroverted uterus.

5. Gently and slowly sound the uterus, which should be between 6 cm and 9 cm.

    a. If sounding less than 6 cm

    b. If sounding greater than 9 cm, stop the insertion due to risk of a perforation; consider repeating the procedure in 2 weeks with consideration of ultrasound guidance and/or referral to a more experienced provider.

6. Load and place IUD according to manufacturer's recommendations for the device (**Figs. 2 and 3**):

    a. ParaGard prescriber's information: https://14wub23xi2gmhufxjmvfmt1d-wpengine.netdna-ssl.com/wp-content/uploads/2018/10/PARAGARD-PI.pdf

    b. Liletta prescriber's information: https://media.allergan.com/actavis/actavis/media/allergan-pdf-documents/product-prescribing/liletta_shi_pi.pdf

    c. Mirena prescriber's information: https://labeling.bayerhealthcare.com/html/products/pi/Mirena_PI.pdf

    d. Kyleena prescriber's information: http://labeling.bayerhealthcare.com/html/products/pi/Kyleena_PI.pdf

    e. Skyla prescriber's information: http://labeling.bayerhealthcare.com/html/products/pi/Skyla_PI.pdf

7. Trim IUD strings with scissors 2 cm to 4 cm from the external os. If the uterine sound has centimeter markings, it may be positioned next to the protruding IUD strings to measure where the strings are trimmed.

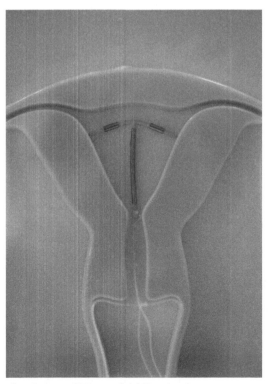

Fig. 2. Model example of copper IUD postinsertion in uterus.

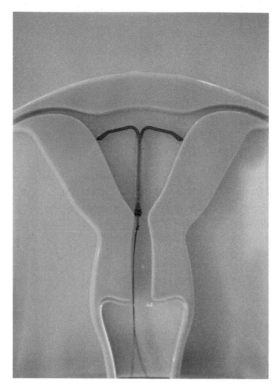

Fig. 3. Model example of an LNG-IUD postinsertion in uterus.

8. Remove tenaculum (if used) and apply pressure using gauze held with the ring forceps to stop any bleeding.
   a. If pressure alone does not achieve hemostasis, silver nitrate or Monsel solution can be applied.
9. Remove speculum.
10. Instruct the patient that she can sit up slowly.
    a. If not dizzy or lightheaded, she may get dressed.
    b. If dizziness or lightheaded, see complications for guidance regarding vasovagal reaction.

ACOG, in conjunction with Innovating Education in Reproductive Health and University of California, San Francisco, Bixby Center for Global Reproductive Health, has created a video series that demonstrates IUD insertion, removal, and common counseling scenarios. The videos are available at https://www.acog.org/programs/long-acting-reversible-contraception-larc/video-series.

RECOVERY AND REHABILITATION

Aftercare and when to call

- Patients often experience uterine cramping after IUD insertion, which can be managed with NSAIDs.
- Nulliparous women are more likely to have increased discomfort with insertion; however, continuation rates are the same as in multiparous women.[33]
- No intercourse or tampon use for 24 hours postinsertion

- Patients should seek immediate attention if they have a positive pregnancy test with an IUD in place, given the likelihood of ectopic pregnancy.

An example patient handout that may be used is from Reproductive Health Access Project: https://www.reproductiveaccess.org/wp-content/uploads/2013/02/iud_aftercare.pdf.

REMOVAL
Discussing Timing for Removal with a Patient

If pregnancy is not desired, removal should be carried out during menstruation, provided the woman still is experiencing regular menses. If removal occurs at other times during the cycle, consider starting a new contraceptive method 1 week prior to removal. If removal occurs at other times during the cycle and the woman has had intercourse in the week prior to removal, she is at risk of pregnancy.

Procedure for Removal

1. Remove IUD by applying gentle traction on the threads with ring forceps.
2. After removal, the system should be examined to ensure that it is intact.
3. If the threads are not visible, determine location of the IUD by ultrasound.
   a. If the IUD is found in the uterine cavity on ultrasound examination, it may be removed with narrow forceps, such as an alligator forceps or an IUD removal hook, which may require dilation of the cervical canal.[34]
   b. If these techniques fail, hysteroscopic removal may be required.

Management

- Complications
  - Difficult insertion: as discussed previously, misoprostol no longer is recommended to help with insertion. If difficult insertion is due to pain, a paracervical block may be useful. If difficult insertion is due to cervical os stenosis, the use of dilators can be considered.[34]
  - Difficult removal: if strings are not immediately visible, twirling a cytobrush placed in the cervical os may trap the strings and pull them into a visible position when it is withdrawn. If this is unsuccessful, ultrasound should be used to confirm intrauterine location of the IUD. If not visible on ultrasound, x-ray imaging should be considered. If the IUD is not intrauterine, referral to gynecologic surgery is indicated. If the IUD is intrauterine, retrieval may be attempted using either an IUD hook or alligator forceps to directly remove the device without the use of strings.[34]
  - Perforation: care should be taken to sound the uterus gently and stop when the fundus is reached. Typically, the uterus should sound to 6 cm to 9 cm.
  - Infection: there is a small risk of intrauterine infection with IUD placement; however, antibiotic prophylaxis is not recommended. STI testing should be performed at time of insertion in those at high risk but does not preclude placing the IUD at the time. If an STI is diagnosed later, treatment can be administered with the IUD in place.[24]
  - Pregnancy: IUD should be removed if a woman becomes pregnant.[24]
  - Vasovagal reaction: may occur with IUD insertion or removal given a patient's anxiety or cervical manipulation, especially if prolonged. Preventive measures include ensuring that patients are hydrated and have eaten before an IUD insertion or removal. Patients who have dizziness or are lightheaded should be kept supine and monitored until symptoms pass. IUD removal may be

helpful if the patient experiences a prolonged episode; however, most patients recover quickly with supportive care.

- Follow-up: instruct the patient to follow-up with her next regularly occurring menstrual cycle to address any concerns of adverse effects and complications.[25]
- Removal: duration of use is conservatively based on manufacturer recommendation; however, the ParaGard, Mirena, and Liletta likely are effective past the manufacturer's recommended removal date. Removal also may be performed at any time if a patient desires return to fertility, is experiencing adverse effects, requests method change, or simply requests removal.

Outcomes

- Pregnancy rate for all FDA-approved IUDs is less than 1% per year.[13]
- Annual rate of adverse events and discontinuation due to side effects is 4.6%.[13]

SUMMARY

IUDs are a safe, effective method of long-term reversible contraception that may be placed in an office-based setting by a qualified provider. IUD placement is simple to perform and has a low complication rate.

CLINICS CARE POINTS

- IUDs are an appropriate form of contraception for most patients, regardless of parity.
- The rate of complication with IUD is relatively low.
- IUDs offer high contraceptive efficacy, with a failure rate of less than 1%.
- Both copper IUDs and the 52-mg LNG IUD (Mirena or Liletta) can be used as emergency contraceptive for 5 days after unprotected intercourse.
- Increasing longevity of efficacy beyond manufacturer's recommendations based on published data
- Ultrasound can assist office-based insertion and removal but usually is not necessary.

DISCLOSURE

S. Long: I am a trainer for the Nexplanon (Merck) implantable contraceptive. I am a trainer for Bayer IUD systems. I am a private stockholder in 1Life Healthcare, which is a publicly traded company.
    L. Colson: nothing to disclose.

REFERENCES

1. Zipper JA, Tatum HJ, Pastene L, et al. Metallic copper as an intrauterine contraceptive adjunct to the "T" device. Am J Obstet Gynecol 1969;105(8):1274–8.
2. Corbett MA. History: the IUD. Reproductive health Access Project; 2013. Accessed January 17, 2021.
3. Margulies L. History of intrauterine devices. Bull N Y Acad Med 1975;51(5):662–7.
4. Burnhill MS. The rise and fall and rise of the IUD. Am J Gynecol Health 1989;(3):6–10.
5. Kaneshiro B, Aeby T. Long-term safety, efficacy, and patient acceptability of the intrauterine Copper T-380A contraceptive device. Int J Womens Health 2010;2: 211–20.

6. Westhoff CL. Current assessment of the use of intrauterine devices. J Nurse Midwifery 1996;41(3):218–23.
7. Available at: https://www.mirena-us.com/. Accessed January 20, 2021.
8. Available at: https://www.paragard.com/. Accessed January 20, 2021.
9. Available at: https://www.skyla-us.com/. Accessed January 20, 2021.
10. Available at: https://www.liletta.com/. Accessed January 20, 2021.
11. Available at: https://www.kyleena-us.com/. Accessed January 20, 2021.
12. Kavanaugh ML, Jerman J. Contraceptive method use in the United States: trends and characteristics between 2008 and 2014. Contraception 2018;97(1):14–21.
13. Ti AJ, Roe AH, Whitehouse KC, et al. Effectiveness and safety of extending intrauterine device duration: a systematic review. Am J Obstet Gynecol 2020;223(1): 24–35.e3.
14. Wu J, Pickle S. Extended use of the intrauterine device: a literature review and recommendations for clinical practice. Contraception 2014;89(6):495–503.
15. McNicholas C, Swor E, Wan L, et al. Prolonged use of the etonogestrel implant and levonorgestrel intrauterine device: 2 years beyond Food and Drug Administration-approved duration. Am J Obstet Gynecol 2017;216(6):586.e1–6.
16. Cheng L, Gulmenzoglu AM, Piaggio G, et al. Interventions for emergency contraception. Cochrane Database Syst Rev 2008;(2):CD001324.
17. Turok D, Gero A, Simmons R, et al. Levonorgestrel vs copper intrauterine devices for emergency contraception. N Engl J Med 2021;384:335–44.
18. CDC. How to be reasonably certain that a woman is not pregnant in: us selected practice recommendations for contraceptive use 2016. Available at: https://www. cdc.gov/reproductivehealth/contraception/ebook.html. Accessed January 28, 2021.
19. Stanback J, Nakintu N, Qureshi Z, et al. Does assessment of signs and symptoms add to the predictive value of an algorithm to rule out pregnancy? J Fam Plann Reprod Health Care 2006;32:27–9.
20. Foster DG, Karasek D, Grossman D, et al. Bimla Schwarz. Interest in using intrauterine contraception when the option of self-removal is provided. Contraception 2012;85(3):257–62.
21. Hubacher D, Chen PL, Park S. Side effects from the copper IUD: do they decrease over time? Contraception 2009;79(5):356–62.
22. Darney P, Stuart G, Thomas M, et al. Amenorrhea rates and predictors during 1 year of levonorgestrel 52 mg intrauterine system. Contraception 2018;97(3): 210–4.
23. ACOG Committee Opinion No. 735: adolescents and long-acting reversible contraception: implants and intrauterine devices. Obstet Gynecol 2018;131(5): e130–9.
24. Hardeman J, Weiss BD. Intrauterine devices: an update. Am Fam Physician 2014;89(6):445–50.
25. Johnson BA. Insertion and removal of intrauterine devices. Am Fam Physician 2005;71(1):95–102.
26. Monif GR, Thompson JL, Stephens HD, et al. Quantitative and qualitative effects of povidone-iodine liquid and gel on the aerobic and anaerobic flora of the female genital tract. Am J Obstet Gynecol 1980;137(4):432–8.
27. Osborne NG, Wright RC. Effect of preoperative scrub on the bacterial flora of the endocervix and vagina. Obstet Gynecol 1977;50(2):148–51.
28. Culligan PJ, Kubik K, Murphy M, et al. A randomized trial that compared povidone iodine and chlorhexidine as antiseptics for vaginal hysterectomy. Am J Obstet Gynecol 2005;192(2):422–5.

29. Meckstroth K, Paul M. First trimester aspiration abortion. In: Paul M, Lichtenberg ES, Borgatta L, et al, editors. Management of unintended and abnormal pregnancy: comprehensive abortion care. John Wiley and Sons; 2009. https://doi.org/10.1002/9781444313031. Available at:.

30. Cason P, Goodman S. Protocol for provision of intrauterine contraception. San Francisco: UCSF Bixby Center Beyond the Pill; 2016.

31. Bluestone J, Chase R, Lu ER. IUD Guidelines for Family Planning Service Programs. USAID. 3rd edition. Baltimore, MD: JHPIEGO; 2006. Available at: https://resources.jhpiego.org/system/files/resources/iud_manual_0.pdf. Accessed January 28, 2021.

32. Eid JF. Penile implant: review of a "No-Touch. Tech Sex Med Rev 2016;4(3): 294–300.

33. Lohr PA, Lyus R, Prager S. Use of intrauterine devices in nulliparous women. Contraception 2017;95(6):529–37.

34. Prine L, Shah M. Long-acting reversible contraception: difficult insertions and re-movals. Am Fam Physician 2018;98(5):304–9.

Contraceptive Implant Insertion and Removal

Bernadatte G. Gilbert, MD[a,b]

KEYWORDS

- Nexplanon • Implantable contraceptive device
- Long-acting reversible contraception

KEY POINTS

- The Nexplanon is a highly effective progestin-only implant exerting contraceptive benefits for up to 3 years.
- It is generally well tolerated with the changes in menstrual bleeding pattern being the most common side effect.
- It can be inserted and removed by a trained health care provider as an office-based procedure with complications being uncommon, especially given the improved applicator design.
- After insertion and confirmation of proper placement, no further monitoring or routine follow-up visits are necessary.

Nexplanon is the only contraceptive implant currently available in the United States. It is a 4 cm × 2 mm rod that contains 68 mg of the progestin etonogestrel. Nexplanon was approved by the Food and Drug Administration in 2011 and differs from its predecessor, Implanon, in several ways: Nexplanon contains barium sulfate, making it radiopaque and allowing more tools to locate a lost implant, and it features an improved applicator design, which minimizes the risks of deep placement and premature loss of the implant from the device. Nexplanon exerts its contraceptive effects by slowly releasing etonogestrel, which suppresses ovulation, increases viscosity of the cervical mucous, and alters the lining of the endometrium leading to endometrial atrophy.

Nexplanon is a form of long-acting reversible contraception (LARC). The unintended pregnancy rate with the implant within the first year of typical use is 0.05%.[1] Like other LARCs, Nexplanon does not require ongoing effort from the patient for its long-term effectiveness. Several professional organizations, including the American College of Obstetricians and Gynecologists and the American Academy of Pediatrics, have endorsed the safety and use of LARCs, to include use in nulliparous persons and

a Department of Family and Community Medicine, Penn State Health Milton S. Hershey Medical Center, 500 University Dr., H154/C1626, Hershey, PA 17033, USA; b Penn State Health Medical Group, Nyes Road Family Practice II, 121 Nyes Road, Suite F, Harrisburg, PA 17112, USA
E-mail address: bgilbert1@pennstatehealth.psu.edu

Prim Care Clin Office Pract 48 (2021) 545–554
https://doi.org/10.1016/j.pop.2021.07.002
0095-4543/21/© 2021 Elsevier Inc. All rights reserved.

adolescents.[2] It is also a useful method for persons with contraindications to, or history of serious adverse reactions from, estrogen.

The implant should be removed by the end of the third year of use. A new implant can be reinserted at the time of removal if continued contraception is wanted. Persons will experience a rapid return to fertility once the implant is removed. By 1 week after removal, circulating levels of etonogestrel are undetectable. Within 3 to 4 weeks of removal, more than 90% of persons will ovulate. In clinical trials of Implanon, pregnancies were observed to occur as early as 7 to 14 days after removal; the same return to fertility is expected with Nexplanon. The implant does not protect against sexually transmitted infections (STIs), and persons should be counseled on methods to reduce acquisition of STIs. For healthy persons, no physical examination or laboratory tests are indicated before insertion, with the exception of a urine pregnancy test. Baseline weight and body mass index measurement may be useful to monitoring implant users for changes over time.

All health care providers must receive manufacturer-specific Nexplanon training before performing insertions or removals of the implant. Training can be requested at https://www.nexplanontraining.com/.

INDICATIONS

Nexplanon is indicated for the use by those with female reproductive pelvic anatomy to prevent pregnancy.

CONTRAINDICATIONS

Nexplanon should not be used in those with female reproductive pelvic anatomy who have the following[3]:

- Known or suspected pregnancy
- Current or past history of thrombosis or thromboembolic disorders
- Liver tumors, benign or malignant, or active liver disease
- Undiagnosed abnormal genital bleeding
- Known or suspected breast cancer, personal history of breast cancer, or other progestin-sensitive cancer, now or in the past
- Allergic reaction to any of the components of Nexplanon

The US Medical Eligibility Criteria for Contraceptive Use classifies implants as a category 2 (**Table 1**) for those with a current or past history of thrombosis or

Table 1 Categories for medical eligibility criteria for contraceptive use	
Category 1	A condition for which there is no restriction for the use of the contraceptive method
Category 2	A condition for which the advantage of using the method generally outweigh the theoretic or proven risks
Category 3	A condition for which the theoretic or proven risks usually outweigh the advantages of using the method
Category 4	A condition that represents an unacceptable health risk if the contraceptive method is used

Data from Curtis KM, Tepper NK, Jatlaoui TC, et al. U.S. Medical Eligibility Criteria for Contraceptive Use, 2016. MMWR Recomm Rep 2016;65(No. RR-3):1–104.

thromboembolic disorders, noting that any increased risk of thromboembolic events is substantially less than that seen with combined oral contraceptives.[1]

ADVERSE REACTIONS

Persons should be counseled regarding adverse reactions they may experience before insertion, allowing persons to know what to expect, as follows:

- Change in menstrual bleeding patterns
  - Change in frequency (absent, less, more frequent, or continuous), intensity (reduced or increased), or duration
  - Range from amenorrhea to frequent and/or prolonged bleeding
  - Bleeding pattern experienced during the first 3 months is predictive of future bleeding pattern
  - Most common reason for discontinuation in clinical studies of Implanon
- Disturbances in liver function
- Emotional lability
- Weight increase
- Headache
- Acne
- Depression
- Vaginitis
- Broken or bent implant

The relative risk of ectopic pregnancy may be increased; however, the absolute risk of ectopic pregnancy is not increased.[2]

DRUG INTERACTIONS

Medications that may decrease the effectiveness of the Nexplanon include barbiturates, griseofulvin, rifampin, phenylbutazone, carbamazepine, felbamate, oxcarbazepine, topiramate, and modafinil. St. John's wort may also reduce its effectiveness.

TIMING OF INSERTION

It is important to rule out pregnancy before inserting Nexplanon. The absence of pregnancy can be reasonably concluded if the person meets any of the criteria in **Box 1**.[4] A pregnancy test at least 2 weeks after the last episode of sexual intercourse is needed when there is doubt. In the situation where a health care provider is unclear whether the person might be pregnant, the benefits of starting the implant likely exceed any risk.[4] Inserting the implant should be considered at any time, with a follow-up pregnancy test in 2 to 4 weeks. There is currently no evidence that the implant will cause abnormal fetal development. Recommendations have been provided in regards to the timing of insertion based on the patient's prior contraceptive use (**Table 2**).

EQUIPMENT

- Examination table
- Sterile drape and gloves
- Antiseptic solution
- Surgical marker
- 1% lidocaine with or without epinephrine
- A One and one-half inch 25- to 27-gauge needle attached to a 5-mL syringe
- Sterile adhesive strip for closure of the puncture site

Box 1
How to be reasonably certain that a person is not pregnant

A health care provider can be reasonably certain that a person is not pregnant if they have no symptoms or signs of pregnancy and meet any one of the following criteria:

- Is ≤7 days after the start of normal menses
- Has not had sexual intercourse since the start of last normal menses
- Has been correctly and consistently using a reliable method of contraception
- Is ≤7 days after spontaneous or induced abortion
- Is within 4 weeks postpartum
- Is fully or nearly fully breastfeeding (exclusively breastfeeding or the vast majority [≥85%] of feeds are breastfeeds), amenorrheic, and less than 6 months postpartum

From Curtis KM, Jatlaoui TC, Tepper NK, et al. U.S. Selected Practice Recommendations for Contraceptive Use, 2016. MMWR Recomm Rep 2016;65(No. RR-4):1–66.

Table 2
Recommend timing of insertion[a]

Previous Contraception Method	Timing of Insertion
No preceding hormonal contraceptive use in the past month	Between day 1 (first day of menstrual bleeding) and day 5 of the menstrual cycle
Combined hormonal contraceptives	Preferably on the day after the last active tablet or on the day of removal of the vaginal ring or transdermal patch; at the latest, on the day following the usual tablet-free, ring-free, patch-free, or placebo tablet interval
Progestin injectable contraceptive	On the day the next injection is due
Progestin-only pill	Any day of the month within 24 h after taking the last tablet
Progestin implant/IUD	On the same day the previous contraceptive is removed
First-trimester pregnancy loss or termination	Within 5 d following pregnancy loss or termination
Second-trimester pregnancy loss or termination	Between 21 and 28 d following pregnancy loss or termination
Postpartum, not breastfeeding[b]	Between 21 and 28 d postpartum
Postpartum, breastfeeding[b]	After the fourth postpartum week

[a] If differing from the recommended timing of insertion, the person should be advised to use a barrier method until 7 d after insertion.
[b] The US Medical Eligibility Criteria for Contraceptive Use classifies implants as a category 2 in breastfeeding postpartum persons at less than 21 d postpartum and 21 to less than 30 d postpartum regardless of their risk for venous thromboembolism (VTE).[1] It classifies implants as a category 1 in breastfeeding postpartum persons at 30 to 42 d postpartum and more than 42 d postpartum regardless of their risk of VTE. For postpartum nonbreastfeeding persons, it classifies implants a category 1 for all scenarios.[1] The implant can be inserted at any time postpartum in breastfeeding and in nonbreastfeeding persons if it is reasonably certain that the person is not pregnant.[4]
Data from NEXPLANON. Package Insert. Merck & Co., Inc.; Revised 11/2020.

- Sterile gauze and elastic pressure bandage
- Sterile no. 11 blade scalpel, forceps (straight and curved mosquito)
- Sterile, preloaded Nexplanon applicator

PROCEDURE

A video can be viewed on the Nexplanon training Web site (https://www. nexplanontraining.com/) for the insertion procedure and removal procedure of palpable implant. Access to these videos is for trained health care providers only. Access is only offered after in-person training has been completed.

Insertion Technique

The correct and carefully performed subdermal insertion of the Nexplanon is the foundation for its successful use and subsequent removal.

1. Obtain informed consent. The completed consent form should be maintained in the patient's medical record.
2. Position the patient. The patient lies on their back on the examination table with the nondominant arm flexed at the elbow and externally rotated. The hand should be located underneath the head or as close as possible to this position (**Fig. 1**A). The clinician should be able to view the applicator from the side to assess the advancement of the needle.
3. Identify the insertion site in the desired (usually nondominant) arm. The insertion site overlies the triceps muscle 8 to 10 cm from the medial epicondyle and 3 to 5 cm below the sulcus (groove) between the biceps and triceps (see **Fig. 1**B). Avoiding the sulcus minimizes risk of insertion into the neurovascular bundle.
4. Using a surgical marker, mark the spot the implant will be inserted. Place a second, guiding mark 5 cm proximal to serve as a directional guide for insertion.
5. Confirm the site is in the correct location. Prepare the skin from the insertion site to the guiding mark with the antiseptic solution of choice and apply sterile drapes.
6. Anesthetize the insertion area with 3 to 5 mL lidocaine with or without epinephrine. Create a wheal where the device needle will enter the skin and then infiltrate along the planned track of the insertion needle.
7. Remove the sterile preloaded disposable NEXPLANON applicator carrying the implant from the packaging.
8. Hold the applicator just above the needle at the textured surface. Remove the transparent protection cover by sliding it away from the needle (see **Fig. 1**C). Confirm the presence of the white-colored implant by looking into the tip of the needle.
9. Do not touch the purple slider until the needle has been fully inserted in a subdermal location. Doing so could retract the needle and prematurely release the implant. If this occurs, restart the procedure with a new applicator.
10. Provide countertraction distally from the insertion site with the free hand (see **Fig. 1**D).
11. Pierce the skin with the tip of the needle angled slightly less than 30° to the skin and insert until the bevel is just under the skin (see **Fig. 1**E).
12. Lower the applicator to a horizontal position and tent the skin by lifting upward as the needle is advanced in its entirety toward the guiding mark (see **Fig. 1**F). Do not exert excessive force if resistance is encountered.
13. Unlock the purple slider by pushing it down slightly. Without moving the applicator, move the slider fully back until it stops (see **Fig. 1**G). Performing this step

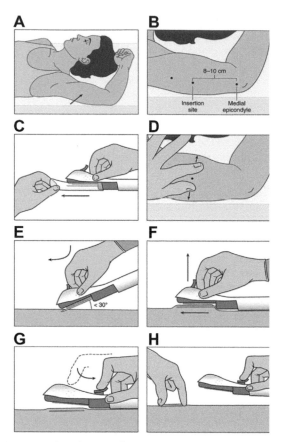

Fig. 1. (*A-H*) Insertion procedure (see text for details). Figures depict the left inner arm. (*From* Grochma SA, Patterson DA. Chapter 136: Insertion and Removal of Nexplanon. In: Fowler GC, ed. Pfenninger & Fowler's Procedures for Primary Care. 4th ed. Elsevier; 2019:948.)

before the needle is fully inserted in the skin will leave a segment of the implant outside the skin and necessitate repeating the procedure with a new device.

14. The implant should now be in place, and the needle is locked into the applicator. Remove the applicator.
15. Verify the presence of the implant by palpating both ends of the implant immediately after insertion (see **Fig. 1**H). If the rod is not palpable, first check the applicator. The needle should be fully retracted, and only the purple tip of the obturator should be visible. If the rod is not identified, use other methods to confirm the presence of the implant. Suitable methods for localization include 2-dimensional x-ray, x-ray computed tomography (CT scan), high-frequency ultrasound, or MRI. If these methods fail, call the Merck National Service Center at 1-877-888-4231.
16. If the presence of the implant is verified by palpation, request that the patient palpate the implant.
17. Apply a sterile adhesive strip to close the puncture wound. Tincture of Benzoin may improve adherence of sterile adhesive strips.
18. Apply a pressure bandage using sterile gauze and elastic pressure bandage. This dressing may be removed in 24 hours.
19. Complete the user card and give the card to the patient.

Complications of Insertion Procedure

- Deep insertion of the implant
- Shallow insertion of the implant
- Partial insertion of the implant
- Unrecognized noninsertion
- Vascular injury
- Local nerve injury
- Postprocedure pain and ecchymosis
- Infection in the insertion area
- Migration of the implant
- Intravascular insertion
- Local irritation or rash
- Expulsion
- Allergic reactions

Removal Technique of an Implant that is Palpable

1. Obtain informed consent. The completed consent form should be maintained in the patient's medical record.
2. Position the patient. The patient lies on their back on the examination table with the arm containing the implant flexed at the elbow and externally rotated. The hand should be located underneath the head or as close as possible (see **Fig.** 1A).
3. Assess the location of the implant with palpation (**Fig.** 2A). Locate the proximal end of the implant and push down to stabilize it. This should allow a bulge to appear, which indicates the distal tip of the implant. Mark the distal tip with a surgical marker.
4. Prepare the skin with the antiseptic solution of choice and apply sterile drapes.
5. Anesthetize the planned incision site with 1 to 2 mL of 1% lidocaine with or without epinephrine. Inject most of the anesthetic deep to the implant to avoid obscuring the implant (see **Fig.** 2B).
6. While stabilizing the proximal end of the implant, make a 2- to 4-mm incision parallel to the implant at the distal tip (see **Fig.** 2C). Use caution to avoid cutting the tip of the implant.
7. Ideally, the tip of the implant will protrude out of the incision. If not, gently push the implant toward the incision until the tip is visible. Blunt dissection of the tissue surrounding the implant may be necessary.
8. Grasp the implant with forceps or hemostats (see **Fig.** 2D). Gently separate adherent tissue from the tip of the implant with additional blunt dissection if needed (see **Fig.** 2E). Remove the implant once freed.
9. Measure the implant to confirm it was removed in its entirety (4 cm). If a partial implant is removed, the remaining piece or pieces should be removed by following the instructions above.
10. A new implant may be inserted immediately after removal of the old device if desired. The new implant can be inserted through the same incision from which the previous implant was removed, provided the site is in the correct location for insertion.
11. Apply a sterile adhesive strip for closure of the incision.
12. Apply a pressure bandage using sterile gauze and elastic pressure bandage; this bandage may be removed in 24 hours.

Complications of Removal Procedure

- Local nerve injury

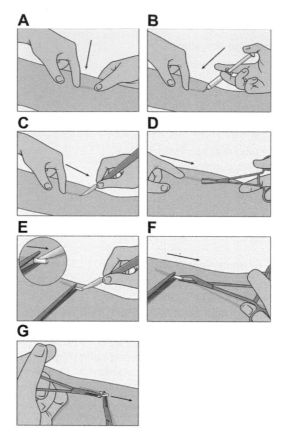

Fig. 2. (*A-G*) Removal procedure (see text for details). Figures depict the left inner arm. (*From* Grochma SA, Patterson DA. Chapter 136: Insertion and Removal of Nexplanon. In: Fowler GC, ed. Pfenninger & Fowler's Procedures for Primary Care. 4th ed. Elsevier; 2019:950.)

- Postprocedure pain and ecchymosis
- Infection in the removal area
- Multiple attempts required
- Broken or bent implant

Localization and Removal of a Nonpalpable Implant

Imaging procedures may be required for location of an implant that is not palpable. Exploratory surgery without knowledge of the exact location of the implant is strongly discouraged.

1. Locate the nonpalpable implant before attempting removal. Suitable methods for localization include 2-dimensional x-ray and x-ray CT. High-frequency ultrasound or MRI may also be used.
2. Remove the implant once it has been localized in the arm. Removal should only be attempted by a health care professional with experience in removing deeply seated implants and who is knowledgeable regarding the anatomy of the arm. Consider use of ultrasound guidance during the removal.
3. Consider applying imaging techniques to the chest if the implant cannot be found in the arm after localization attempts. If the implant is located in the chest, surgical or

endovascular procedures may be needed for removal, and the appropriate health care professional should be consulted.
4. Removal may require a minor surgical procedure or a surgical procedure in an operating room if the implant migrates within the arm. If so, the appropriate health care professional should be consulted.
5. If at any time imaging methods fail to locate the implant, call the Merck National Service Center at 1-877-888-4231 for details on etonogestrel blood level determination.

MONITORING AND FOLLOW-UP

After insertion and confirmation of proper placement of the implant, no further monitoring is necessary, and a routine follow-up visit is not required. For postprocedural pain, over-the-counter analgesics, such as acetaminophen or ibuprofen, are acceptable. Persons should be advised to return at any time to discuss adverse reactions or other concerns, if they have a desire to switch contraception, or for removal of the implant. Health care providers seeing implant users should assess the person's satisfaction and any changes in health status that would change the appropriateness of the implant for safe and effective use.

ONLINE RESOURCES FOR PATIENTS AND CLINICIANS

American College of Obstetricians and Gynecologist Long-Acting Reversible Contraception Program https://www.acog.org/programs/long-acting-reversible-contraception-larc.
  Clinical Training Program for Nexplanon https://www.nexplanontraining.com/
  Nexplanon Patient Education https://www.organonconnect.com/nexplanon/patient-education/
  Nexplanon Professional Resources https://www.organonconnect.com/nexplanon/professional-resources/
  Patient Web site for Nexplanon https://www.nexplanon.com/
  Reproductive Health Access Project https://www.reproductiveaccess.org/contraception/

CLINICS CARE POINTS

- When inserting the Nexplanon, care should be taken to correctly identify the insertion site (overlying the triceps muscle about 8–10 cm from the medical epicondyle of the humerus and 3–5 cm below the sulcus between the biceps and triceps muscle) to avoid the large blood vessels and nerves that lie within and around the sulcus.

- When inserting the Nexplanon, caution should be exercised to avoid deep insertion, which can lead to difficulty in palpating the Nexplanon and impede the removal process.

- Immediately following insertion, verify the presence of the implant by palpation. If unable to palpate the device, steps should be taken to confirm correct placement.

DISCLOSURE

No disclosures.

REFERENCES

1. Curtis KM, Tepper NK, Jatlaoui TC, et al. U.S. medical eligibility criteria for contraceptive use, 2016. MMWR Recomm Rep 2016;65(No.RR-3):1–104.

2. American College of Obstetricians and Gynecologists. Long acting reversible contraception: implants and intrauterine devices. ACOG Practice Bulletin No. 186. Obstet Gynecol 2017;130(5):e251–69.
3. NEXPLANON [package insert]. Whitehouse Station, NJ: N.V. Organon, Oss, The Netherlands, a subsidiary of Merck & Co., Inc; 2020.
4. Curtis KM, Tepper NK, Jatlaoui TC, et al. U.S. selected practice recommendations for contraceptive use, 2016. MMWR Recomm Rep 2016;65(No.4):1–66.

Endometrial Biopsy
Indications and Technique

Stephanie Long, MD[a,b]

KEYWORDS

- Endometrial biopsy • Abnormal uterine bleeding • Premenopausal
- Postmenopausal

KEY POINTS

- Abnormal uterine bleeding is a frequent medical concern for premenopausal and post-menopausal patients
- Endometrial biopsy is a safe, cost-effective option that is offered in the office setting
- Complications from endometrial biopsy are low
- Topical cervical analgesia and oral NSAIDs, such as ibuprofen, can decrease a patient's discomfort during an endometrial biopsy

INTRODUCTION

Abnormal uterine bleeding (AUB) accounts for a significant number of ambulatory care visits.[1] An endometrial biopsy is an easy procedure to offer in the office setting to aid in the evaluation and diagnosis of abnormal and postmenopausal uterine bleeding. Providing access in the outpatient primary care setting provides patients with timely evaluation for potentially serious medical conditions.

Uterine and endometrial cancers have been increasing in incidence and mortality in the United States.[2] The greatest increase in uterine and endometrial cancers has been in non-Hispanic Black and Asian women.[3] However, as Cote and colleagues[3] note in their study, "for nearly every stage and subtype, the 5-year relative survival for [non-Hispanic Black] women is significantly less than [non-Hispanic white] women, whereas Hispanic and Asian women have the same or better survival." Although providers must continue to research the cause for the increase, particular attention needs to be paid to address these significant racial disparities.

An endometrial biopsy is an initial test to look for abnormal uterine cells. It is a procedure during which a sample of the endometrial tissue is obtained using a small sampling device that is inserted into the uterus to sample cells of the uterine body. The tissue obtained is examined by a pathologist and used to guide treatment or additional diagnostic work-up.

---

[a] University of Washington, Department of Family Medicine, Seattle, WA, USA; [b] Family Medicine Residency of Idaho, 777 North Raymond Street, Boise, ID 83704, USA
E-mail address: Stephanie.long@fmridaho.org

Prim Care Clin Office Pract 48 (2021) 555–567
https://doi.org/10.1016/j.pop.2021.07.003
0095-4543/21/© 2021 Elsevier Inc. All rights reserved.

DEFINITIONS

AUB is a large diagnostic category that encompasses a significant change to the amount, frequency, duration, or timing of bleeding during or between periods.

Postmenopausal bleeding is bleeding that occurs after a period of menstrual cessation that is equal to or greater than 12 months. Postmenopausal bleeding warrants prompt evaluation.

INDICATIONS
Abnormal Uterine Bleeding

Endometrial malignancy or hyperplasia is one possible diagnosis for AUB. The International Federation of Gynecology and Obstetrics has classified nine different diagnoses that may cause uterine bleeding and comprise a comprehensive differential diagnosis list.[4] They are remembered with the help of the mnemonic PALM COEIN: polyp, adenomyosis, leiomyoma, malignancy and hyperplasia, coagulopathy, ovulatory dysfunction, endometrial, iatrogenic, and not otherwise specified. Iatrogenic reasons may be caused by medications, such as gonadal steroids and tamoxifen. Not otherwise specified etiologies encompass such entities as arteriovenous malformations or endometriosis.

Risk factors for endometrial cancer include "age, obesity, use of unopposed estrogen, specific medical comorbidities (eg, polycystic ovary syndrome, type 2 diabetes mellitus, atypical glandular cells on screening cervical cytology), and family history of gynecologic malignancy."[5]

An endometrial biopsy can help identify the presence of malignancy or hyperplasia of the uterus by sampling the tissue and allowing for examination by a pathologist. It may aid in ruling in or out a diagnosis while pursuing additional work-up. It may also assist in the monitoring of a previously identified uterine abnormality.

Postmenopausal Bleeding

Bleeding that occurs after menopause warrants evaluation to evaluate for endometrial precancerous changes or neoplasia.

Abnormal Pathology on Cervical Cancer Screening Assessment

An endometrial biopsy may be indicated from the results of a cervical cancer screening Pap smear. This may be done before or as part of a colposcopy. Per the 2019 American Society for Colposcopy and Cervical Pathology Consensus guidelines "Endometrial sampling is recommended in conjunction with colposcopy and endocervical sampling in nonpregnant patients 35 years or older with all categories of AGC and AIS. Endometrial sampling is also recommended for nonpregnant patients younger than 35 years at increased risk of endometrial neoplasia based on clinical indications (eg, AUB, conditions suggesting chronic anovulation, or obesity)."[6]

Indications for an endometrial biopsy are summarized in **Box 1**.

CONTRAINDICATIONS

- Pregnancy
- Acute vaginitis, cervicitis, or pelvic inflammatory disease
- Cervical cancer
- Coagulopathy is a relative contraindication. Some conditions may be appropriate for an office procedure. However, more significant or symptomatic disease may preclude an outpatient procedure.

Box 1
Indications for endometrial biopsy at a glance

- Abnormal uterine bleeding
- Postmenopausal bleeding
- Surveillance for previously diagnosed endometrial neoplasia or precancerous hyperplasia
- Abnormal findings on cervical Pap smear
  - Atypical glandular cells
  - Endometrial cells
    - May be normal or abnormal in appearance and warrant evaluation (eg, normal endometrial cells are abnormal in the postmenopausal patient)

ALTERNATIVES

- Expectant management with possible delayed and/or missed diagnosis of potentially threatening disease.
- Imaging may provide additional information about the endometrial lining or an alternative diagnosis.
  - Transvaginal ultrasonography is a reasonable alternative to endometrial sampling as a first approach in evaluating a postmenopausal woman with an initial episode of bleeding. If blind sampling does not reveal endometrial hyperplasia or malignancy, further testing, such as hysteroscopy with dilation and curettage, is warranted in the evaluation of women with persistent or recurrent bleeding.
  - In patients with postmenopausal uterine bleeding, transvaginal ultrasound revealing an endometrial thickness of 4 mm or less has a greater than 99% negative predictive value for endometrial cancer.[5]
- Dilation and curettage/uterine aspiration.
- Guided biopsy via hysterosalpingogram.

RISKS

- Inability to perform the procedure because of several factors, such as:
  - Patient intolerance of an office-based examination and procedure because of anxiety or pain.
  - Stenotic cervix that prevents entry to the uterus.
- Insufficient tissue obtained
  - An endometrial biopsy is a blind sampling of the uterine lining. Excess blood may mean that the blood to cell ratio is too high for the pathologist to have sufficient cells to examine. Inadequate sampling may also result in insufficient tissue.
  - About 11% of biopsies do not produce any tissue for examination.[7]
- Diagnostic errors
  - False-negative results are possible. Endometrial biopsy is 90% sensitive for endometrial cancer and 82% sensitive for atypical hyperplasia. If there are persistent symptoms or other concerns, additional or repeat evaluation is advised.
  - Specificity approaches 100% for postmenopausal and premenopausal patients.[7,8]
- Infection
  - There is a low risk of infection when using sterile instruments and appropriate technique.

- Uterine perforation
  - Uncommon; the risk is likely no greater than with comparable intrauterine procedures, such as intrauterine device, at 0.1% to 0.3%.[9]

BENEFITS

- Endometrial biopsy is an office-based procedure, thereby increasing access and facilitating scheduling without additional risks of anesthesia or the cost of operating room
- Pathology review and diagnosis that informs a patient treatment plan
- Helps identify the need for additional studies, including diagnostic imaging or diagnostic procedures, such as a hysterosalpingogram

PREPARATION
Trauma-Informed Care

Many patients have experienced physical, emotional, or sexual trauma in their lives. Health care experiences can compound preexisting trauma or be a source of trauma themselves. A patient need not disclose a specific history of trauma for medical care to be provided in a trauma-informed matter.

In a 2001 publication, Harris and Fallot[10] outline five core values for trauma-informed care that aid health care providers in approaching patients: (1) safety, (2) trustworthiness, (3) choice, (4) collaboration, and (5) empowerment. Patients must be assured of their physical and emotional safety when engaging in medical care. There should be clear expectations about the course of their experience. Offering options and patient control where applicable facilitates patient engagement and empowerment. Patients become active agents in their care and share power when care is approached through a trauma-informed lens.[11–13]

Informed Consent

The indications, risks, benefits, and alternatives for the procedure should be thoroughly discussed with the patient before the procedure. Aftercare instructions and next steps after the biopsy should be reviewed.

Some patients may find it helpful to see the collection device and/or a demonstration of an endometrial biopsy. Any uterine model can assist with this process as shown in **Fig. 1**.

To support transparency and collaboration, it may be important to review with patients that there are two parts to the endometrial biopsy. There is the office-based procedure called the endometrial biopsy and a pathology examination of the endometrial sample. Frequently these are two separate charges for patients: one originating from the office and another from the laboratory.

Patient Comfort

Pharmacotherapy

- Pain management and anxiolytics are of benefit
  - Preprocedure nonsteroidal anti-inflammatory drugs (NSAIDs), such as ibuprofen, are recommended to assist with cramping.
  - There are little data that opioids improve pain scores during intrauterine procedures. However, they do increase the risks given their effects on sedation and airway. Little data support the use of opioid-containing medications currently.

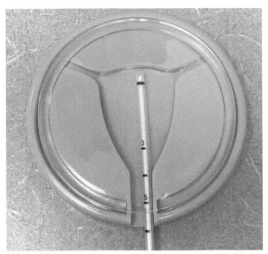

Fig. 1. Patient demonstration of an endometrial biopsy with a uterine model and nonsterile endometrial biopsy suction device. Note that it may be helpful to label any demonstration equipment "Not for patient use."

- o Anxiolytics may be beneficial for some patients. However, benefit must be weighed against risks of medications and any considerations for airway support and monitoring in the office.
- o Several investigations are underway for other options, such as gabapentin, for patient comfort during intrauterine procedures.
- Cervical preparation with misoprostol is not recommended
  - o Misoprostol may increase side effects (nausea, cramping) without impacting success of the procedure across premenopausal and postmenopausal patients.[14,15]
  - o If a failed first attempt is caused by cervical stenosis, misoprostol may be considered.

Nonpharmacologic considerations

- Heating pad or disposable heat pack
- Support individual
- Distraction with music, guided imagery
- Several investigations are underway exploring such options as transcutaneous electrical nerve stimulation and acupuncture

Equipment List

- Nonsterile gloves (**Figs. 2–8**)
- Sterile gloves
- Gauze and/or scopettes
- Scissors (if planning to cut and submit catheter tip with biopsy specimen)
- Ring forceps
- Cervical tenaculum
- Speculum
- Uterine sound, plastic or metal
- Formalin container with patient label
- 10% Lidocaine spray or 2% gel

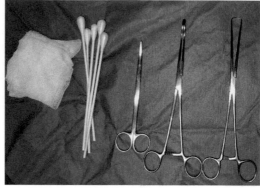

Fig. 2. Sterile equipment laid out on sterile lining with from left to right sterile gauze, scopettes, scissors, ring forceps, and cervical tenaculum.

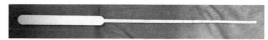

Fig. 3. Plastic disposable uterine sound removed from sterile packaging.

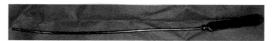

Fig. 4. Metal reusable uterine sound removed from sterile pouch.

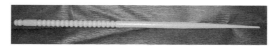

Fig. 5. Disposable plastic cervical os finder removed from sterile packaging.

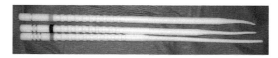

Fig. 6. Reusable sterile cervical os finders with varying tapered ends removed from sterile pouch.

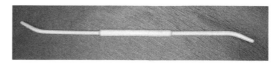

Fig. 7. Plastic reusable cervical dilator. Typically only the smallest dilator is necessary as shown here removed from sterile pouch.

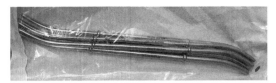

Fig. 8. Metal reusable cervical dilator. Typically only the smallest dilator is necessary to pass an endometrial sampling device. However, many providers may have dilators as a set in a single sterile pouch as pictured here.

- Patient drape
- Endometrial biopsy collection device
  - Pipelle Endometrial Suction Curette (https://coopersurgical.com/detail/pipelle-endometrial-suction-curette)
  - Wallach Endocell Disposable Endometrial Cell Sample (https://coopersurgical.com/detail/wallach-endocell-disposable-endometrial-cell-sampler)
  - Endosampler by Gynex (https://gynexcorporation/product/endosampler)
  - Manual vacuum aspirator using a small cannula (https://hpsrx.com/MVA-products)
    - Providers may have this device onsite because it is used in clinic aspiration or suction procedures for early pregnancy loss and early abortions
- May consider:
  - Chlorohexidine or povidone-iodine solution
  - Cervical os finder, disposable or reusable, if needed
  - Cervical dilators, if needed
  - Underwear liner or sanitary pad (or patients may be instructed to bring their own)

PROCEDURE TECHNIQUES
Trauma-Informed Care

- Using the principles of trauma-informed care may decrease the trauma of medical experiences and patient anxiety. In the steps of the procedure outlined later, there are also suggestions for patient engagement and trust-building during the endometrial biopsy.

No Touch Sterile Technique

- Regardless of when sterile gloves are used during an endometrial biopsy, it is possible to contaminate equipment. It is common to use a "no touch technique" whereby no equipment that enters the uterus is touched.[16]

Cervical Cleaning

- Cervical cleaning with an aseptic solution has been a traditional step for intrauterine procedures. There is little evidence to support the need for this step to reduce infection and many have eliminated this step.
- Chlorhexidine is preferred over povidone-iodine if including an aseptic solution.[17–19]

Personal Protective Equipment

- Collection is not an aerosolizing procedure regardless of which sampling device is used.
- Some providers may wear safety glasses or a face shield to prevent accidental mucous membrane exposure to bloody body fluids.

- If using a paracervical or intracervical block, ensure that the needle is disposed of in an appropriate safety container.
- Not all waste produced requires biohazard waste destruction. Ensure that regular and biohazard disposal receptacles are available.

PROCEDURE STEPS

1. Patient positioning and draping.
   a. Dorsal lithotomy with use of knee or footrests.
   b. Paper or cloth drapes may be used to minimize unnecessary patient exposure.
2. Request permission and receive consent from the patient to begin the examination.
3. Perform a bimanual examination to assess the uterine position and size.
4. Insert the speculum to visualize the cervix.
   a. Consider offering the patient the opportunity to insert the speculum or assist with the insertion.
5. Cervical anesthesia should be used.
   a. Topical application with a product, such as lidocaine spray or gel, reduces patient discomfort.
   b. Intracervical lidocaine gel is associated with reduced pain during endometrial biopsy.[20–35]
      i. Intracervical 2% lidocaine gel for 3 minutes before biopsy is appropriate.
   c. Paracervical or intracervical block may be used for patient comfort.
6. Apply the tenaculum to the cervix.
   a. Most commonly this is applied to the anterior lip of the cervix at 12 o'clock.
   b. However, posterior placement may be helpful for a retroverted uterus.
   c. In addition, tenaculum may be applied to the left or right side of the cervix in an anterior-posterior orientation if this assists in performing the procedure.
7. Sound the uterus.
   a. Typical sounding depth is 6 to 8 cm.
   b. If sounding shallow at less than 6 cm, sample may be collected in the cervix and be inadequate. In addition, uterine fibroids or changes to uterine anatomy may result in shallow sounding.
   c. If sounding deep at greater than 9 cm, perforation is a consideration.
      i. If perforation is suspected, abort the procedure.
      ii. If an ultrasound is available, consider reattempting with ultrasound guidance. Otherwise, it is possible to reattempt after 2 weeks with consideration of ultrasound guidance and/or referral to a more experienced provider.
8. Cervical dilation may be necessary to sound and/or pass the sampling device.
   a. Cervical os finders can be used.
   b. Small plastic or metal cervical dilators may also be helpful.
9. Some providers change to sterile gloves at this point in the procedure.
   a. It is still necessary to maintain "no touch technique" for any equipment that enters the uterus.
10. Insert the collection catheter into the uterus.
11. Withdraw the internal piston (or pull back on the syringe plunger) to create suction.
12. Rotate the device 360° while moving the tip back and forth in the endometrial cavity from fundus to internal os.
13. Once the sampler is full of tissue, remove the collection device and deposit the tissue in the formalin container for transfer to the laboratory.
    a. An additional pass may be necessary to collect an adequate sample.

b. Some providers using a Pipelle or Endocell collector cut off the tip (1–2 cm) and submit to the laboratory because additional cells may collect in the rounded ended of the collection device.
14. Remove the equipment slowly after notifying the patient the procedure has finished.
15. Observe the tenaculum site and external os for significant bleeding.
    a. Pressure with a scopette or gauze may be necessary to stop bleeding.
    b. Occasionally silver nitrate or Monsel solution may be needed for tenaculum site hemostasis.
16. Patient recovery.
    a. Intense cramping often subsides quickly.
    b. Patients should get up slowly after the procedure. If dizzy or lightheaded, recommend the patient lie down until symptoms resolve.
    c. Light bleeding or spotting is expected, and an underwear liner or sanitary pad can be offered.

AFTERCARE INSTRUCTIONS

Aftercare instructions should be part of preprocedure planning so a patient can know what to expect in advance. Many patients benefit from receiving aftercare instructions in their own language. They are provided with a printout or electronic instructions via a patient portal. An example of aftercare instructions is provided in **Box 2**.

Box 2
After your endometrial biopsy patient instructions example

After Your Endometrial Biopsy

It is normal to have some mild cramping for a few days after the procedure. Ibuprofen (ie, Advil) is recommended to help manage cramps. Acetaminophen (Tylenol) may be less effective for cramps but can be used in addition to ibuprofen or in place of it.

You may want to have someone drive you home from the office on the day of your procedure. This may be required if you have any sedatives during the procedure.

You will have light bleeding for 1 to 2 days after the procedure. You may want to wear a liner or sanitary pad for bleeding.

Your provider may recommend not to place anything in the vagina for 2 to 3 days after an endometrial biopsy to decrease the risk of bleeding and/or infection. This includes douching, tampons or menstrual cup, or anything that may be inserted during sex (hands, penis, or toys).

You may return to your normal activities. However, if you find that you are having increased bleeding then you may want to avoid strenuous activity or heavy lifting.

Your provider will make a plan with you for communicating test results and discussing next steps.

Call your health care provider if you have any of the following:

• Excessive bleeding, such as passing clots or bleeding longer than 2 days after the procedure

• Foul-smelling discharge from your vagina

• Fever or chills or feel unwell

• Severe lower abdominal pain

• If you have any concerns and want assistance

COMPLICATIONS

- Unable to perform the procedure
  - Cervical stenosis may be present in postmenopausal patients or in postsurgical patients, most commonly in those who have undergone a loop electrocautery excision procedure.
  - Misoprostol preprocedure may be of benefit. Cervical os finder, cervical dilators, or lacrimal dilators may be helpful to gain initial access to the external os.
  - Ultrasound guidance may be helpful if difficult to pass through the cervix or challenging anatomy.
- Insufficient tissue
  - If the cause was not from inability to complete or attempt the procedure, then repeat sampling in the office or referral for sampling with hysterosalpingogram are options guided by patient preference, cost, and/or other logistics.
- Patient discomfort
  - Cramping, pain, and patient anxiety are managed with the techniques and medications outlined previously. Occasionally, they may be a reason that the patient or provider believes it is necessary to terminate the attempted procedure.
- Vasovagal reaction
  - Can be common with cervical and intrauterine procedures. Most resolve spontaneously.
- Bleeding
  - Often minimal and controlled with pressure alone.
  - Cervical bleeding may require application of silver nitrate or Monsel solution for hemostasis.
  - More significant uterine or cervical bleeding is rare but should be handled as an emergency with office-based care and/or referral to a more experienced provider or hospital location.
  - Laceration at the cervical tenaculum site may rarely require suturing to stop brisk bleeding.
- Infection
  - Uncommon.
  - If patients develop signs or symptoms of endometritis, they should be treated promptly with appropriate antibiotic therapy.
- Perforation
  - If cervical or uterine perforation is suspected, the procedure should be aborted.
  - Reattempt under ultrasound guidance and/or referral to a more experienced provider is recommended.
  - If a perforation is suspected, observe the patient until no longer symptomatic or refer if persistently symptomatic.

DISCUSSION

Providers should make a plan with the patient to discuss and review results and/or next steps. Some patients may desire an office, telephone, or virtual visit. Others may opt for an electronic portal message or letter to allow time for an emotional response before they have a discussion with their provider. It may help to ask how a patient might want to receive information about a cancer diagnosis to better inform the follow-up plan. Other patients may not want to discuss possible results in advance for cultural or personal beliefs. Respecting a patient's decision about how and when to receive information is an important part of their care.

For interpretation of results, it is best practice to consult up-to-date resources from the major societies. The next steps may be informed by a patient's medical history, other diagnostic information, age, and/or risk factors.

SUMMARY

Endometrial biopsy is a tool that aids in the diagnosis of abnormal and postmenopausal uterine bleeding. The procedure is performed safely in the office. Preprocedure NSAIDs and topical cervical anesthesia decrease patient discomfort during the biopsy. Trauma-informed care may increase patient engagement in the decision to proceed with recommended medical care and their perception of their experience.

CLINICS CARE POINTS

- Abnormal uterine bleeding is a frequent medical concern for premenopausal and postmenopausal patients.
- Endometrial biopsy is a safe, cost-effective option that is performed in the office setting.
- Complications from endometrial biopsy are low.
- Topical cervical analgesia and oral NSAIDs, such as ibuprofen, can decrease a patient's discomfort during an endometrial biopsy.
- Routine cervical preparation with misoprostol is not recommended.
- Although there are a variety of sampling devices to collect an endometrial biopsy, they all function by insertion of a catheter into the uterus, which creates gentle suction in the collection device that removes tissue.
- Rotating the device 360° while moving the tip back and forth in the endometrial cavity from fundus to internal os facilitates collection of an appropriate sample. Some providers may perform a second pass to ensure adequate tissue.
- Endometrial biopsy is 90% sensitive for endometrial cancer, 82% sensitive for atypical hyperplasia, and 100% specific for premenopausal and postmenopausal patients.

DISCLOSURE

The author is a private stockholder in 1Life Healthcare, which is a publicly traded company; a trainer for Merck's Nexplanon implantable contraceptive; and a trainer for Bayer's IUD systems.

ACKNOWLEDGMENTS

Loren Colson, DO, with whom I worked on the Intrauterine Device Insertion and Removal article. The sources for cervical cleansing, no touch technique, and complications were obtained as part of the literature search for our joint publication. I thank my prior teachers and mentors who helped instruct me on the art of practicing patient-centered care. I express gratitude to the countless patients who have trusted me as a partner in their health care journey. They have provided feedback that has allowed me to become the physician and teacher that I am today.

REFERENCES

1. Spencer CP, Whitehead MI. Endometrial assessment revisited. Br J Obstet Gynaecol 1999;106:623–32.

2. Cronin KA, Lake AJ, Scott S, et al. Annual report to the nation on the status of cancer. Part I: national cancer statistics. Cancer 2018;124:2785–800.

3. Cote ML, Ruterbusch JJ, Olson SH, et al. The growing burden of endometrial cancer: a major racial disparity affecting black women. Cancer Epidemiol Biomarkers Prev 2015;24:1407–15.

4. Munro G, Critchley HO, Broder MS, et al. FIGO classification system (PALM-COEIN) for causes of abnormal uterine bleeding in nongravid women of reproductive age. Int J Gynaecol Obstet 2011;113(1):3–13.

5. ACOG committee opinion No. 734 summary: the role of transvaginal ultrasonography in evaluating the endometrium of women with postmenopausal bleeding. Obstet Gynecol 2018;131:945–6.

6. Perkins R, Guido R, Castle P, et al. 2019 ASCCP risk-based management consensus guidelines for abnormal cervical cancer screening tests and cancer precursors J. Low Genit Tract Dis 2020;24(2):102–31.

7. van Hanegem N, Prins MM, Bongers MY, et al. The accuracy of endometrial sampling in women with postmenopausal bleeding: a systematic review and meta-analysis. Eur J Obstet Gynecol Reprod Biol 2016;197:147–55.

8. Dijkhuizen FP, Mol BW, Brölmann HA, et al. The accuracy of endometrial sampling in the diagnosis of patients with endometrial carcinoma and hyperplasia: a meta-analysis. Cancer 2000;89(8):1765–72.

9. Johnson BA. Insertion and removal of intrauterine devices. Am Fam Physician 2005;71(1):95–102.

10. Harris M, Fallot R. Using trauma theory to design service systems. San Francisco: Jossey-Bass; 2001.

11. Reeves E. Synthesis of the literature on trauma-informed care. Issues Ment Health Nurs 2015;36(9):698–709.

12. Guarino K, Soares P, Konnath K, et al. Trauma-informed organizational toolkit. Rockville, MD: Center for Mental Health Services; 2009.

13. Wilson C, Pence D, Conradi L. Trauma-informed care. In: Encyclopedia of social work. From Oxford Press and National Association of Social Workers Press; 2013. Available at: https://oxfordre.com/socialwork/view/10.1093/acrefore/9780199975839.001.0001/acrefore-9780199975839-e-1063. Accessed January 31 2021.

14. Crane JMG, Craig C, Dawson L, et al. Randomized trial of oral misoprostol before endometrial biopsy. J Obstet Gynaecol Can 2009;31(11):1054–9.

15. Perrone JF, Caldito G, Mailhes JB, et al. Oral misoprostol before office endometrial biopsy. Obstet Gynecol 2002;99(3):439–44.

16. Meckstroth K, Paul M. First trimester aspiration abortion. In: Paul M, Lichtenberg ES, Borgatta L, et al, editors. Management of unintended and abnormal pregnancy: comprehensive abortion care. John Wiley and Sons; 2009.

17. Monif GR, Thompson JL, Stephens HD, et al. Quantitative and qualitative effects of povidone-iodine liquid and gel on the aerobic and anaerobic flora of the female genital tract. Am J Obstet Gynecol 1980;137(4):432–8.

18. Osborne NG, Wright RC. Effect of preoperative scrub on the bacterial flora of the endocervix and vagina. Obstet Gynecol 1977;50(2):148–51.

19. Culligan PJ, Kubik K, Murphy M, et al. A randomized trial that compared povidone iodine and chlorhexidine as antiseptics for vaginal hysterectomy. Am J Obstet Gynecol 2005;192(2):422–5.

20. Karaca I, Yapca OE, Adiyeke M, et al. Effect of cervical lidocaine gel for pain relief in Pipelle endometrial sampling. Eurasian J Med 2016;48(3):189–91.

21. Einarsson JI, Henao G, Young AE. Topical analgesia for endometrial biopsy: a randomized controlled trial. Obstet Gynecol 2005;106(1):128–30.
22. Aksoy H, Aksoy U, Ozyurt S, et al. Effect of lidocaine spray in pain management during office-based endometrial sampling: a randomized placebo-controlled trial. J Obstet Gynaecol 2016;36(2):246–50.
23. Luangtangvarodom W, Pongrojpaw D, Chanthasenanont A, et al. The efficacy of lidocaine spray in pain relief during outpatient-endometrial sampling: a randomized placebo-controlled trial. Pain Res Treat 2018;2018:1238627.
24. US Cancer Statistics Working Group. United States cancer statistics: 1999–2015 cancer incidence and mortality data. Atlanta, GA: US Department of Health and Human Services; 2018. Available at: https://www.cdc.gov/cancer/npcr/uscs/index.htm. Accessed December 28 2020.
25. Null DB, Weiland CM, Camlibel AR. Postmenopausal bleeding: first steps in the workup. J Fam Pract 2012;61:597–604.
26. Braun M, Overbeek-Wager E, Grumbo R. Diagnosis and management of endometrial cancer. Am Fam Physician 2016;93(6):468–74.
27. ACOG Committee Opinion no 631 summary: endometrial interaepithelial neoplasia. Obstet Gynecol 2015;125(5):1272–1278l.
28. ACOG Practice bulletin no. 128: diagnosis of abnormal uterine bleeding in reproductive-aged women. Obstet Gynecol 2012;120(1):197–206.
29. ACOG committee opinion no. 557: management of acute abnormal uterine bleeding in nonpregnant reproductive-aged women. Obstet Gynecol 2013;121(4):891–6.
30. Narice BF, Delaney B, Dickson JM. Endometrial sampling in low-risk patients with abnormal uterine bleeding: a systematic review and meta-synthesis. BMC Fam Pract 2018;19(1):135.
31. Vilos GA, Lefebvre G, Graves GR. Guidelines for the management of abnormal uterine bleeding. J Obstet Gynecol Can 2001;23(8):704–9.
32. Raja S, Hasnain M, Hoersch M, et al. Trauma informed care in medicine: current knowledge and future research directions. Fam Community Health 2015;38(3):216–26.
33. Williams P, Gaddey H. Endometrial biopsy: tips and pitfalls. Am Fam Physician 2020;101(9):551–6.
34. Somchit W, Lertkhachonsuk AA, Vallipakorn SA. Naproxen for pain relief during endometrial biopsy: a randomized controlled trial. J Med Assoc Thai 2015;98(7):631–5.
35. Zuber T. Endometrial biopsy. Am Fam Physician 2001;63(6):1131–5.

Bartholin Gland Abscess Diagnosis and Office Management

Natalie Long, MD*, Laquita Morris, MD, Krystal Foster, MD

KEYWORDS

- Bartholin gland abscess • Word catheter • Marsupialization

KEY POINTS

- Word catheter or Jacobi ring catheter placement should be offered as an initial treatment to individuals with a first episode of Bartholin gland abscess.
- While Word catheters and Jacobi ring catheters have similar complication and recurrence rates, the Jacobi ring catheter has the advantages of being less likely to dislodge prematurely and higher patient satisfaction.
- In the absence of overlying cellulitis or systemic infection, antibiotics are unnecessary for management of Bartholin gland abscess when surgical drainage is performed.
- Depending on practitioner experience and preference, marsupialization may be performed in the management of primary or recurrent Bartholin gland abscesses in the outpatient setting.
- Surgical excision is reserved for refractory cases and should not be performed if active infection is present.

INTRODUCTION

The Bartholin glands are pea sized and located bilaterally at the 4 and 8 o'clock positions of the labia minora. They drain through 2.0 to 2.5 cm long ducts, allowing for vaginal lubrication during intercourse and sexual arousal.[1] They may also help with keeping moisture over the surface of the vulva.[2] These ducts can become obstructed by trauma, mucus, or edema, causing cyst formation. Cysts are most commonly located in the lower third of the vagina, between the vestibule and labium minora.[2] Smaller cysts can be asymptomatic. Abscesses may protrude anteriorly and grow to be 5 to 8 cm in diameter.[2] Bartholin gland abscesses are more often due to secondary infection of an existing cyst than a primary infection.[3] Bartholin gland abscesses are three times more commonly diagnosed than cysts and predominantly affect younger women. Although rare, malignancy of the Bartholin gland can occur most commonly in postmenopausal women and should be excluded in women aged older than 40 years with biopsy or excision.[1]

Department of Family and Community Medicine, University of Missouri, Columbia, M224 Medical Sciences Building, DC032.00, Columbia, MO 65212, USA
* Corresponding author.
E-mail address: longna@health.missouri.edu

Prim Care Clin Office Pract 48 (2021) 569–582
https://doi.org/10.1016/j.pop.2021.07.013
0095-4543/21/© 2021 Elsevier Inc. All rights reserved.

primarycare.theclinics.com

NATURE OF THE PROBLEM

Bartholin gland cysts and abscesses may affect between 2% and 3% of women.[3] Bartholin gland cysts most commonly arise gradually, over several weeks or months, are often unilateral, and may be asymptomatic if small. Abscesses can be distinguished from cysts as they often arise over the course of days, are painful, are associated with medially protruding vulvar edema, and may have overlying erythema or fluctuance. Active purulent drainage may also be present at the time of presentation.[2] Vulvar pain can occur with walking, sitting, or intercourse. Recognition and treatment of Bartholin gland abscesses can decrease the patient's risk for sepsis, need for antibiotic therapy, and hospitalization.[3,4]

Risk factors for Bartholin gland cysts and abscesses are similar to risk factors for sexually transmitted infections and include single women, women with multiple sexual partners, and lower socioeconomic status.[2–4] More than 80% of isolates are mixed vaginal flora, and the most common include *Bacteroides spp.*, *Escherichia coli*, and *Staphylococcus aureus*.[4] *Streptococcus pneumonia* and *Haemophilus influenzae* are becoming more common, likely due to oral sex practices.[1] Routine testing for sexually transmitted infections should be ordered for patients presenting with Bartholin gland abscesses, although *Gonorrhea* and/or *Chlamydia* are rarely isolated.[4] Antibiotics should be reserved for cases with associated cellulitis of the overlying skin or systemic involvement.[2–4]

Other vulvar pathologies may appear similarly to Bartholin gland cysts and abscesses. Sebaceous cysts can be found within the labia majora and are commonly superficial. Near the mons, folliculitis may be appreciated, commonly associated with *S aureus* infection. In the case of folliculitis, pustules appear to be more common than abscesses and require antibiotic use only. Other vulvar ducts may become obstructed as well, causing cyst or abscess formation, including Gartner's duct and Skene's gland. The Gartner's duct is located on the lateral wall, and Skene's gland is located on the anterior wall of the vulva. Given their proximity to the urethra, abscesses may be associated with urethral obstruction and urinary retention. Hidradenitis suppurativa has a predilection for genital skin and can be found more commonly in patients with higher levels of melanin in the skin.[1]

Bartholin gland abscesses diagnosed during pregnancy require immediate surgical intervention and drainage to avoid severe infection or pregnancy complications. The preferred method of treatment during pregnancy is unclear. Similar to nonpregnant patients, the most common pathogen is *E coli*.[5]

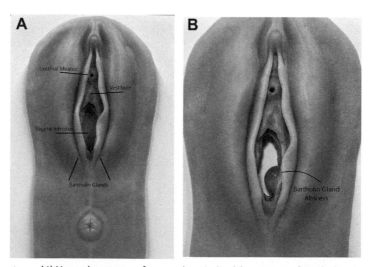

Fig. 1. Anatomy. (*A*) Normal anatomy of external genitalia. (*B*) Anatomy of Bartholin gland abscess.

ANATOMY (FIG. 1)
Management

Outpatient management consists of incision and drainage (I&D) followed by either fistulization using a Word catheter or Jacobi ring catheter or destruction using silver nitrate, alcohol, or CO2 laser. Marsupialization may be performed in the outpatient setting using local anesthesia, though depending on practitioner experience and resources, some may prefer the operating room with regional anesthesia. Total cyst excision may be required for recurrent episodes and is best performed in the operating room. Treatment can be based on patient preferences, local resources, and practitioner experience and expertise. Beginning with I&D with Word catheter placement has advantages that include acceptable recurrence rates and the ability to be performed in an outpatient setting.[3] Simple I&D should be avoided as recurrence rates are high. Recurrence can occur after fistulization or destruction, ranging from 2.7% to 17.4%; therefore, women should be counseled that subsequent therapy may be necessary.[3] Many infections are polymicrobial, and antibiotics are indicated when surrounding erythema or systemic involvement is present.[2–4]

Simple incision and drainage
I&D alone offers simplicity with shorter treatment time and faster healing than more invasive techniques. However, due to high rates of recurrence, simple I&D is no longer commonly used for Bartholin gland abscess treatment.[1]

Fistulization
The first-line treatment for an abscess of the Bartholin's gland is incision, drainage, and insertion of a Word catheter.[3,6] Word catheters are short rubber tubes measuring around 5 cm. The tip of the catheter has a small balloon that can hold up to 3 mL of saline.[2] After I&D, the Word catheter is placed into the abscess cavity, and the balloon is inflated. The catheter remains in place for 4 weeks.[7] Owing to the presence of the foreign body, wound closure is prevented, allowing for reepithelialization of the outflow tract.[1] Patients may benefit from Word catheter placement by avoiding general anesthesia and need for hospitalization.[1]

Alternatively, a Jacobi ring catheter may be inserted. While not commercially sold, it can be crafted out of either 8 French or butterfly tubing threaded with a 2-0 suture. Following the creation of a tunnel through the cyst cavity, the tubing is drawn through the cyst, and the suture is tied, creating a loop that remains in place for 3 to 4 weeks.[8,9] Ring catheters have similar recurrence rates to Word catheters but are less likely to dislodge prematurely.[1,8,9] Patient satisfaction is similar but was reported to be higher with ring catheter placement in one small study.[9]

Destruction
Alcohol sclerotherapy or silver nitrate application is an alternative method of treatment that leads to destruction of the epithelial lining of the Bartholin gland cyst or abscess. Following aspiration or drainage of the cyst, the destructive element is inserted. Main risks include discomfort, labial edema, and tissue necrosis. Both methods have similar tolerability and complication rates, although healing times are longer with silver nitrate application.[10] CO_2 laser destruction or excision has also been reported, though the cost and operator expertise are limiting factors in

utilization of this technique. After using the laser to create an opening in the skin overlying the cyst, the contents of the cyst are evacuated and the vaporized, excised, or left intact after fenestration.[4]

Marsupialization

Marsupialization is often preferred if the patient has a latex allergy because the stem of the standard Word catheter is latex, although silicone-based catheters are also now available. Marsupialization or excision may also be preferred if the patient has had a recurrence after one or two trials at Word catheter placement or has a larger abscess greater than 5 cm.[1,11] The goal of marsupialization is to create a surgical pouch by suturing the cyst capsule to the excision edge. This prevents closure of the excision and allows for duct patency and ongoing drainage of the cyst, eventually resulting in reepithelization of the tract.[2] A linear incision the length of the cyst wall is made on the medial aspect of the abscess and distal to the hymenal ring.[2] Using interrupted absorbable sutures on a small needle, the cyst wall and mucosa are sutured to the external edge of the incision.[1]

Excision

Full excision of the gland is not recommended during active infection. In refractory cases, such as multiple recurrences and failed conservative measures, excision can be considered.[2] Common complications include vaginal dryness, hemorrhage or hematoma (2%–8%), and dyspareunia (8%–16%).[2,4] Though vaginal dryness may occur, removal of a Bartholin gland does not usually affect lubrication due to the presence of other glands, including the Skene glands.[1] Excisions are typically performed in the operating room by a gynecologist. Recurrence rates are low (0%–3%), and healing time ranges from 9 to 12 days.[4] (**Box 1**) and (**Box 2**).

Box 1
Preprocedure planning for fistulization, destruction, or marsupialization

Written informed consent is obtained before the procedure. A discussion about risks, benefits, and alternatives to the procedure is held with the patient, and any questions about the procedure should be addressed.

Equipment preparation
- Sterile gloves
  - Face shield or mask and eyewear
  - Betadine solution
  - 4 × 4 sterile gauze
  - 1% to 2% lidocaine, with or without epinephrine
  - 25g needle with 5 mL syringe
- 11 blade
- Hemostat
- Adjustable light source
- Disposable pad to place under patient's hips

Procedural steps[1,12]
1. Patient is placed into lithotomy position
2. Sterile gloves, eyewear, and mask or face shield should be donned by the provider
3. Cleanse perineum with povidone iodine solution
4. Identify abscess and evert the labia majora for better visualization
5. Anesthetize the subdermal area overlying the abscess with 1% or 2% lidocaine, with or without epinephrine

Pro Tip: Avoid injecting lidocaine into the cyst cavity to prevent premature drainage or explosive decompression at the time of incision.

Box 2
Pudendal nerve block (optional, but may be required for adequate anesthesia before marsupialization)

Risks: local anesthetic toxicity related to large doses of anesthesia, hematoma, or abscess formation

Benefits: up to 1 hour of pain relief

Procedure: Inject 5 to 10 mL of 1% lidocaine through the vaginal side wall directed toward the ischial spine on side of body with abscess using Iowa trumpet and 20-gauge needle. Be sure to aspirate syringe before injecting local anesthetic to prevent intravascular injection

Data from Schrock SD, Harraway-Smith C. Labor analgesia. *Am Fam Physician*. 2012;85(5):447-454.

Word catheter placement

Equipment preparation (**Figs. 2** and **3**)
- #11 blade
- Sterile saline
- Word catheter
- 18g needle with 3 mL syringe
  - Adson forceps

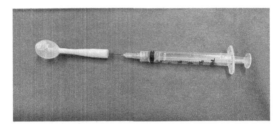

Fig. 2. Word catheter.

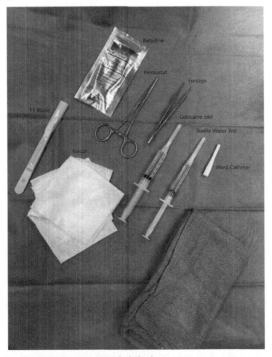

Fig. 3. Word catheter equipment tray with labels.

- Hemostat

Procedural steps[1,7,12,13] (**Fig. 4**)

Following adequate local anesthesia,

1. The wall of the abscess may be grasped with small forceps for better manipulation
2. A small 3- to 5-mm stab incision is created with a #11 blade distal to hymenal ring and interior to the labium minora

    Pro Tip: A hemostat can be placed next to the blade within the incision to break up any loculations present and to grasp the abscess wall for accurate catheter placement
3. Manual expression of the abscess encourages drainage
4. Flush the area with sterile saline

    Pro Tip: Test for leakage of the catheter bulb before insertion by inflating it with 3 mL of saline solution using the needle and syringe
5. Place the Word catheter through the stab incision
6. Using the 3 mL syringe and 18g needle, inflate the bulb of the catheter with 3 mL of sterile saline

    Pro Tip: Keep pressure on plunger while withdrawing needle to avoid backfilling syringe before creation of vacuum seal
7. The tail of the catheter can be tucked into the vaginal canal for patient comfort

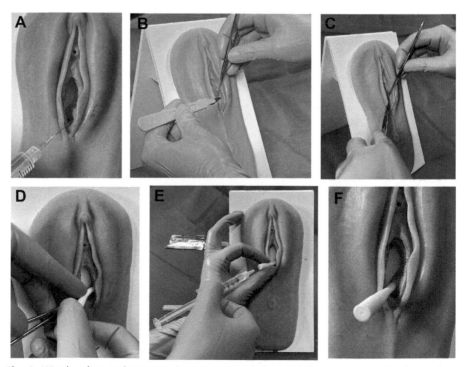

Fig. 4. Word catheter placement demonstration. (*A*) Inject lidocaine around the base of abscess or cyst. (*B*) Make 5 mm incision just distal to the hymenal ring. (*C*) Insert an hemostat to aid with drainage and break up any loculations present. (*D*) Insert the Word catheter into the cyst cavity. (*E*) Inflate the Word catheter with 3 mL of sterile water. (*F*) Word catheter remains in place for 4 weeks. End may be tucked into the vagina for patient comfort.

Jacobi Ring placement

Equipment preparation (**Figs. 5** and **6**)
- #11 blade
- Tubing/catheter (either 8 French T tube cut to 7 cm or Butterfly tubing cut to 5 cm)
- A 2-0 silk suture trimmed to 20 cm and threaded through tubing
- Curved hemostat
    Pro Tip: Silk suture will thread through tubing more easily than nylon suture.

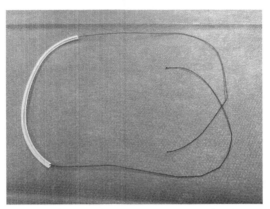

Fig. 5. Jacobi Ring. A Jacobi Ring is made by trimming 8 French tube or Butterfly tubing to 5 to 7 cm length. Thread with 20 cm of 2-0 or 3-0 silk suture.

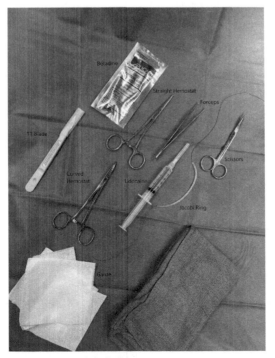

Fig. 6. Jacobi ring equipment tray labeled.

Procedural steps[1,8,9] (**Fig. 7**)
Following adequate local anesthesia,
1. Using 11 blade, make 3-5 mm incision distal to the hymenal ring and interior to the labium minora
2. Using curved hemostat, pass into abscess tunneling upward and back to vaginal mucosa
3. Make 2nd incision at the tip of the hemostat, allowing the end to protrude
4. Grasp the end of the catheter/tubing that has been threaded with the suture
5. Pull the catheter/tubing back through the tunnel taking care not to pull the suture out
6. Once the end emerges, tie suture ends together forming a closed ring.

Postprocedural care and follow-up instructions following fistulization

Before patient discharge, ensure that the patient has access to proper analgesia.

Following Word catheter placement, follow-up should be scheduled 1 week post-procedure to assess patient tolerance and to confirm that the catheter remains in place. The time for reepithelialization varies from patient to patient and can occur between 2 and 3 weeks. After about 4 weeks, or once reepithelialization is complete, the patient should return for catheter removal. By deflating the balloon, the catheter can be removed without anesthesia.[7]

Following Jacobi ring placement, follow-up is scheduled in 3 weeks for catheter removal following reepithelialization.[9] After cutting the suture, the tubing can be gently withdrawn[8] (**Box 3**).

Box 3
Sexual activity following fistulization

In 2015, Reif and colleagues[14] studied the effects of treatment with a Word catheter on quality of life and sexual activity. About 81% of their study population reported continuation of sexual activity while the Word catheter remained in place. Although the study participants did not explicitly clarify whether sexual activity included vaginal penetration, the participants denied discomfort during sexual activity with Word catheter treatment. Although women are often counseled to avoid sexual activity immediately following fistulization procedures, many women do remain sexually active without serious complications while the device is in place.[14]

Alcohol sclerotherapy

Equipment preparation
- 18g needle with 10 cc syringe
- 10 mL alcohol 70%
- Additional 10 cc syringe
- Hemostat

Procedural steps[10]
After adequate local anesthesia,
1. Identify point of maximum fluctuations
2. Insert 18g needle with an attached syringe
3. Aspirate the cyst completely
4. Remove the syringe containing cyst contents and replace with the syringe filled with alcohol
   Pro Tip: Keep the needle within the cyst cavity during exchange
5. Use a similar volume of alcohol 70% to what was aspirated from the cyst

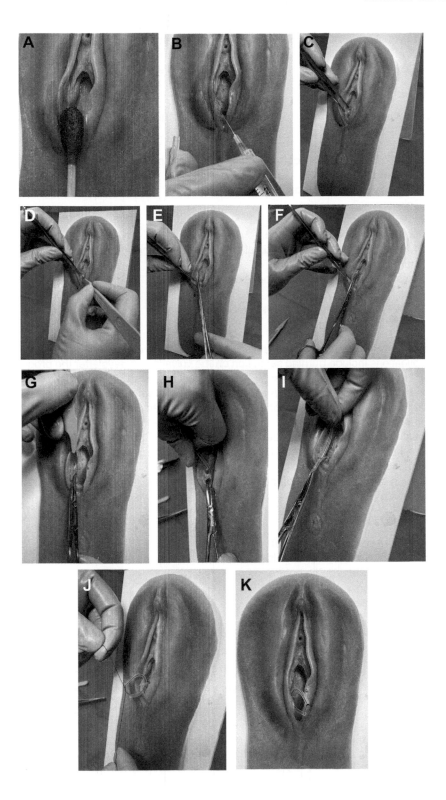

6. Inject alcohol 70% into the cyst cavity and irrigate continuously for 5 minutes
7. End by evacuating the cyst as completely as possible
8. Compress the cyst for several minutes to assure hemostasis

Silver nitrate

Equipment preparation
- #11 blade
- Hemostat
- Silver nitrate stick (typically 2 mm diameter) trimmed to 0.5 cm length
- Needle driver
- Nonabsorbable 4 to 0 or 5 to 0 suture
- Scissors

Procedural steps[10]
After adequate local anesthesia,
1. Make 1-2 cm incision just distal to the hymenal ring and interior to the labium minora
2. Use the hemostat to grasp/penetrate the cyst wall
3. Fully drain the cyst
4. Insert trimmed silver nitrate stick into the cavity
5. Close incision with a suture

Postprocedural care and follow-up instructions for destruction techniques

Complications include burning sensation on the vulva in first days after the procedure, labial edema, and ecchymosis as well as tissue necrosis. Scar tissue can result. Sitz baths are recommended to decrease edema. Avoid intercourse for 2 weeks after the procedure, although complication rates are likely low as detailed in **Box 3**.[10]

For silver nitrate application, the patient should follow-up in 3 days for suture removal and to remove necrotized contents of the cyst. After removing the suture, insert a hemostat to grasp the silver nitrate stick and necrotized tissue and withdraw through incision site.[10]

No long-term pain or dyspareunia was reported in a single study using alcohol sclerotherapy.[10]

Marsupialization

Equipment preparation (**Fig. 8**)
- Number 11 or 15 blade scalpel
- 2-0 or 3-0 absorbable suture
- Marking pen
- Needle driver
- Forceps x 2
- Scissors

Fig. 7. Jacobi ring catheter placement demonstration. (*A*) Cleanse area with povidone iodine. (*B*) Inject lidocaine around the base of abscess. (*C*) Grasp the cyst to evert labium minora. (*D*) Make 5 mm incision just distal to the hymenal ring interior to the labium minora. (*E*) Insert a curved hemostat to drain abscess and break up loculations. (*F*) Tunnel curved hemostat upward through cyst cavity. (*G*) Make second 3-5 mm incision. (*H*) Grasp end of tubing. (*I*). Taking care not to dislodge the suture, pull the Jacobi ring back through cyst the cavity. (*J*) Tie the suture together to secure the Jacobi ring. (*K*) Jacobi ring remains in place for 3 to 4 weeks.

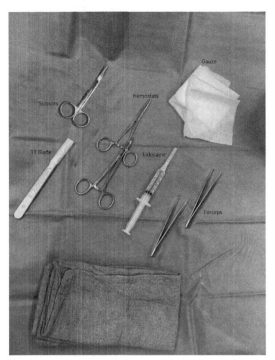

Fig. 8. Marsupialization equipment tray.

- Small hemostat x 2
- Collection tubes for cultures (bacterial, chlamydia and gonorrhea if desired)
- Sterile drapes
- Ribbon gauze (optional for temporary packing if extra bleeding)

Procedural steps[1,2,4,11,15]

Following adequate local anesthesia,

1. Make a 2 to 3 cm incision (length of the cyst wall) over the medial aspect of the abscess distal to the hymenal ring right inside the introitus to minimize scarring and allow drainage of secretions in the vagina, or alternatively, excise an elliptical portion of the vestibular skin and cyst wall in this same location
   a. Consider outlining area for incision (linear vs elliptical) with a marking pen while palpating the cyst location
   b. Incision/excision should not include external labial skin
   c. Incision will traverse internal labial skin, fascia overlying the cyst, vaginal side wall smooth muscles, and cyst capsule
2. Empty the cyst/abscess and break up loculations if needed, consider a sample for culture
3. Irrigate with saline
4. If difficulty with hemostasis, consider temporary packing with ribbon gauze
5. Suture the cyst wall to skin incision edges to prevent closure of incision and reformation of abscess using interrupted absorbable sutures (eg, 2–0 or 3–0 Vicryl with a small needle)

Postprocedural care and follow-up instructions

Patients should be instructed to use sitz baths at least daily beginning on postoperative day 1. Patients should monitor for worsening pain, bleeding, and signs of infection.

Schedule for follow-up in 1 week to ensure healing and again at 4 to 6 weeks.[1,6] Wound healing is expected within 2 weeks.[4]

Outcomes

Aspiration or drainage alone heals quickly but with recurrence rates of up to 38% should be avoided as primary treatment.[1,3,4]

With Word catheter placement, patients may experience vulvar pain, bleeding risk, and the premature expulsion of the Word catheter (before completion of reepithelization).[4] Though at acceptable rates, abscess recurrence may occur with the Word catheter as well, with studies showing 3% recurrence at 6 months and 12% at 12 months.[1] Complications following Jacobi ring placement are comparable to Word catheter placement with the benefit of fewer episodes of premature displacement. Most heal within 3 weeks.[4]

While silver nitrate application has the benefit of quick procedure time (less than 15 minutes) and low recurrence rates of less than 4%, patients report a high frequency of local side effects of labial discomfort and edema. Accidental cautery to vaginal

Table 1 Advantages and disadvantages of treatment modalities for Bartholin's gland abscess		
Procedure	**Advantages**	**Disadvantages**
Simple I&D	Shorter procedure time Immediate relief of discomfort Decreased healing time	High recurrence rate
Word Catheter	Acceptable short-term recurrence rate Low cost No sexual restrictions during treatment	Risk of premature loss of catheter Contraindicated with latex allergy[a]
Jacobi Ring Catheter	Similar to Word catheter Higher patient satisfaction than Word catheter Easy to place	Two incision sites are created Practitioners may not be familiar with technique
Alcohol sclerotherapy	Shorter procedure time	High rate of tissue necrosis and scarring Hematoma may result
Silver Nitrate Ablation	Shorter procedure time Low recurrence rate Less scarring than alcohol sclerotherapy	Frequent reports of labial burning and edema postprocedure Hematoma may result
CO2 Destruction	Shorter procedure time	High cost of laser Operator experience dependent Presence of scar tissue Moderate recurrence rate
Marsupialization	Low recurrence rates	Longer procedure time Longer healing time May require operating room and general anesthesia
Excision	Useful with recurrence or suspected malignancy Infrequent recurrence	Performed in the operating room Persistent dyspareunia Fever

[a] Unless using silicon-based Word catheter now available.
Data from Refs.[1,3,4,12]

mucosa was common, though healing was usually completed within 10 days. Hemorrhage can occur in 4% to 5%.[4] Following alcohol sclerotherapy, recurrence rates are moderate at 8% to 10%, and hematoma formation is more commonly seen, affecting up to 20% of cases. Additionally tissue necrosis and scarring are frequent complications in 17% of patients.[4]

In many of the studies regarding marsupialization, most procedures were performed in the operating room for the use of spinal, epidural, or general anesthesia, though some have been performed in the office setting with local anesthesia or pudendal block.[2–4,6,11] The most common complications following marsupialization include pain, hematoma formation, prolonged healing and draining, secondary infection, scarring, and dyspareunia.[1,2] Based on a randomized controlled study comparing Word catheter placement to marsupialization, marsupialization appears to be less painful (2/10 vs 6.2/10 maximal pain) during the actual treatment itself but did require more frequent analgesic medication in the 24 hours after treatment (73.9% vs 33.3%). However, marsupialization in this study was performed most commonly under spinal or general anesthesia in the operating room. At 1 week, pain scores were similar.[6] Recurrence rates are low, ranging from 5% to 15%.[15] Recurrence was not statistically significant between marsupialization and Word catheter (10.3 vs 12.2%, respectively, 95% CI: 0.64–1.91) at 1 year.[6] The median healing time is approximately 2 weeks.[4]

Following surgical excision, recurrence rates are low (0%–3%). Most heal in 9 to 12 days. Bleeding and hematoma formation are common complications occurring between 2% to 8% of cases. Postoperatively, fever is reported in 24% of cases, and persistent dyspareunia is seen in 8% to 16% of cases[4] (**Table 1**).

SUMMARY

Bartholin gland abscesses are a common outpatient gynecologic concern. Procedural management is key to expedited treatment and recovery. The ideal treatment option requires a brief, safe procedure that is performed in an outpatient setting with local anesthesia and is associated with a low rate of recurrence with fast healing times.[4] While additional studies are required to determine the optimal initial mode of therapy, fistulization, most commonly with Word catheters, is considered first-line treatment. The introduction of Jacobi ring catheters has provided an alternative mechanism for reepithelization that may have advantages over Word catheter placement, including increased patient satisfaction and lack of premature displacement. Methods that lead to cyst cavity destruction are alternatives, though patients report more labial edema and discomfort postoperatively. Marsupialization may require additional anesthesia and operating time, as well as prolonged healing, which make it a less feasible first-line therapy. Excision should be avoided during the initial treatment of a Bartholin gland abscess.

CLINICS CARE POINTS

- During anesthesia, avoid injecting lidocaine directly into the abscess to prevent premature drainage or explosive drainage at the time of incision.
- Consider Jacobi rings for treatment of first Bartholin gland abscess. Be sure to use a silk suture to thread more easily.
- When placing a Word catheter, always remember to check if the catheter inflates well before placing it and keep back pressure on the syringe until the needle is removed to prevent loss of fluid from the catheter.

- Biopsy is recommended in women aged older than 40 years or if Bartholin gland abscess is not improving as expected.

ACKNOWLEDGMENTS

Special thanks to the MU Shelden Clinical Simulation Center, especially Damon Coyle and Dena Higbee, for their assistance with the creation of the task trainers used for demonstrations and photos.

DISCLOSURE

The authors have nothing to disclose.

REFERENCES

1. Omole F, Kelsey RC, Phillips K, et al. Bartholin duct cyst and gland abscess: Office management. Am Fam Physician 2019;99(12):760–6.
2. Bora SA, Condous G. Bartholin's, vulval and perineal abscesses. Best Pract Res Clin Obstet Gynaecol 2009;23(5):661–6.
3. Illingworth BJG, Stocking K, Showell M, et al. Evaluation of treatments for Bartholin's cyst or abscess: a systematic review. BJOG 2020;127(6):671–8.
4. Wechter ME, Wu JM, Marzano D, et al. Management of Bartholin Duct Cysts. Obstet Gynaecol Surv 2009;64(6):395–404.
5. Boujenah J, Le SNV, Benbara A, et al. Bartholin gland abscess during pregnancy: Report on 40 patients. Eur J Obstet Gynecol Reprod Biol 2017;212:65–8.
6. Kroese JA, van der Velde M, Morssink LP, et al. Word catheter and marsupialisation in women with a cyst or abscess of the Bartholin gland (WoMan-trial): a randomised clinical trial. BJOG An Int J Obstet Gynaecol 2017;124(2):243–9.
7. Nohuz E, Lamblin G, Lebail-carval K, et al. Minimally invasive management of Bartholin gland abscesses (with demonstrative video). J Gynecol Obstet Hum Reprod 2020;49(7):1–5.
8. Kushnir VA, Mosquera C. Novel Technique for Management of Bartholin Gland Cysts and Abscesses. J Emerg Med 2009;36(4):388–90.
9. Gennis P, Siu FL, Provataris J, et al. Jacobi ring catheter treatment of Bartholin's abscesses [13]. Am J Emerg Med 2005;23(3):414–5.
10. Kafali H, Yurtseven S, Ozardali I. Aspiration and alcohol sclerotherapy: A novel method for management of Bartholin's cyst or abscess. Eur J Obstet Gynecol Reprod Biol 2004;112(1):98–101.
11. Dole DM, Nypaver C. Management of Bartholin Duct Cysts and Gland Abscesses. J Midwifery Womens Heal 2019;64(3):337–43.
12. Jr EJM, Cooper D. Vu l v a r P ro c e d u re s Biopsy, Bartholin Abscess Treatment , and Condyloma Treatment. Obstet Gynecol Clin North Am 2021;40(4):759–72.
13. Reif P, Ulrich D, Bjelic-Radisic V, et al. Management of Bartholin's cyst and abscess using the Word catheter: Implementation, recurrence rates and costs. Eur J Obstet Gynecol Reprod Biol 2015;190(2015):81–4.
14. Reif P, Elsayed H, Ulrich D, et al. Quality of life and sexual activity during treatment of Bartholin's cyst or abscess with a Word catheter. Eur J Obstet Gynecol Reprod Biol 2015;190(2015):76–80.
15. Omole F, Simmons BJ, Hacker Y. Management of Bartholin's Duct Cyst and Gland Abscess. Am Fam Physician 2003;68(1):135–40.

Management of Cervical Dysplasia Using Office Loop Electrosurgical Excision Procedure

Sarah Inés Ramírez, MD, FAAFP*, Andrew Lutzkanin, MD, FAAFP

KEYWORDS

- Loop electrosurgical excision procedure (LEEP) • Cervical cancer
- Cervical intraepithelial neoplasia (CIN) • Cervical dysplasia

KEY POINTS

- In the United States, excisional treatment (eg, LEEP) is preferred over ablative therapy as the treatment of HSIL.
- The advantages of LEEP are that it allows for complete excision of a cervical lesion, allows for blended cutting, and can be performed in the outpatient setting.
- LEEP should be avoided in the setting of pregnancy, bleeding disorder, infection of the cervix, inability to obtain clear margins, and/or visible malignancy at the time of colposcopy.
- The most common complication after the LEEP procedure is mild bleeding which can last up to 10 days; bleeding maybe heavier in up to 6% of women.
- The risk of preterm birth after the LEEP procedure is similar to that seen with other excisional procedures of the cervix.

INTRODUCTION

While cervical cancer is among the 5 most common gynecologic cancers in the United States (US), it is not among the top 10 causes of cancer-related death, largely due to early detection and treatment of premalignant disease.[1] The US has seen a 70% reduction in the prevalence of human papillomavirus (HPV)-related cervical cancer since the introduction of the HPV vaccine in 2006.[2] High-grade cervical lesions require excision for definitive diagnosis and management as it only takes several years for high-grade lesions to progress to invasive cervical cancer. The loop electrosurgical excision procedure (LEEP) is used to excise cervical lesions using a thin, loop-shaped wire that is heated with electrical current.

Department of Family and Community Medicine, Penn State Health Hershey Medical Center, 500 University Drive, Mail Code HP11, Hershey, PA, USA
* Corresponding author.
E-mail address: sramirez2@pennstatehealth.psu.edu

Prim Care Clin Office Pract 48 (2021) 583–595
https://doi.org/10.1016/j.pop.2021.07.008
0095-4543/21/© 2021 Elsevier Inc. All rights reserved.

primarycare.theclinics.com

Background

Before the advent of LEEP, the traditional treatment for cervical intraepithelial neoplasia (CIN) was conization—surgical removal of a cone-shaped portion of cervical tissue—and/or hysterectomy. In the 1970s, the development of colposcopy allowed for improved precision in the identification and treatment of CIN lesions in a more conservative manner using electrocautery, cryotherapy, and laser ablation. These approaches were largely abandoned in the 1990s with the introduction of LEEP. While not clearly evidence-based, clinicians were increasingly concerned that the older procedures undertreated occult invasive cancer.[3,4]

Advantages

LEEP offers several advantages over other ablative and excisional procedures:[5,6]

- Blended cutting: a combination of both cutting and coagulation electric currents allows for better control of bleeding during and after the procedure.
- Lower cost
  - LEEP can be performed in the office rather than in the operating room.
  - "See and treat:" Patients can be diagnosed and treated in the same visit.
  - Less expensive equipment than laser-based devices.
  - Fewer complications, decreasing downstream cost.
- The entire lesion can be removed and adequately evaluated histologically.[7–9]

Effectiveness

LEEP is highly effective; up to 95% of CIN lesions are completely eradicated with a single treatment.[10–13] One systematic review of 19 studies found a 5.3% risk of recurrence of CIN 2 or CIN 3 at 12 months after LEEP.[14] LEEP is as effective as cold knife excision and has the additional benefit of less tissue loss.

Epidemiology

Prevalence

- Ninety-one percent of cervical cancers are caused by the HPV.[15]
- The highest prevalence of cervical cancer is in women aged 40 - 49 years.[16]
- Between 2008 and 2016, the rate of CIN2+ (CIN2 and CIN3 collectively) declined among women aged 18 to 24 years but increased among women aged 40 to 64 years. Of the 196,000 cases of CIN2+ diagnosed during that time, almost 40% were in women aged 18 to 39 years.[17]
- Approximately 500,000 LEEP procedures are performed in the US annually.[18]
- Persistence of HPV (HPV detected at the first clinical examination after excision procedure) is associated with an 8% rate of recurrent high-grade disease 5 years after LEEP.[19]

Incidence

- In 2016, an estimated 196,000 CIN2+ cases were diagnosed.[17]
- In 2017, nearly 13,000 new cases of cervical cancer were diagnosed, representing 7.5 per 100,000 women.[16]
- In the US, Hispanic women have the highest incidence of cervical cancer.[16]
- The incidence of cervical cancer is highest in women aged 40 - 44 years.[16]

Mortality

- A total of 4207 women died of cervical cancer in 2017.[16]

- When compared to all races, African-American women have the highest rate of death from cervical cancer.[16]
- Women aged 85 years and older have the highest rate of death from cervical cancer.[16]

Definitions

- Papanicolaou smear (Pap smear) of cervix: screening test that samples endocervical and exocervical cells from the squamocolumnar area of the cervix and prepares the cells in a variety of manners for cytologic evaluation in a laboratory.
- Colposcopy: procedure using a binocular microscope (colposcope) to directly visualize the cervix. Stains and chemicals are used to evaluate for the presence of cellular dysplasia, vascular, and tissue abnormalities.
- Endocervical curettage (ECC): the use of an endocervical curette to obtain a sample of tissue from the endocervical canal.
- "Top Hat" LEEP: a two-step procedure that uses the conventional LEEP followed by a second excision of the residual endocervix using a smaller-diameter loop.
- Cold knife cone (CKC) biopsy (cervical conization): deep excision of the cervical transformation zone using a laser or scalpel.
- Atypical squamous cells (ASCs) of undetermined significance: the most commonly reported cervical cytology finding. Most commonly, ASC represents a benign reactive process, but up to 10% of cases may harbor high-grade squamous intraepithelial lesion.[20]
- Atypical glandular cells (AGCs) represent either endocervical, endometrial, or not otherwise specified lesions.[21] While AGC accounts for less than 0.8% of cytologic findings on Pap smear, up to 50% may have findings of CIN, adenocarcinoma in situ, or adenocarcinoma.[22]
- CIN: a precancerous condition in which abnormal cells grow on the surface of the cervix.
- Abnormal changes of the cervical epithelium (**Fig. 1**) are described using the Bethesda Classification System (**Table 1**).

Anatomy

The uterine cervix connects the uterus and the upper portion of the vagina. Its structure is made up of an external and internal opening (os) connected by an endocervical canal measuring approximately 3 cm in length. The endocervical canal is lined by columnar epithelium, while the surface of the cervix most adjacent to the vagina is lined by stratified squamous epithelium. The interface of the two cell types is termed the squamocolumnar junction. The transformation zone represents an area where columnar epithelium transforms into squamous epithelium; the transformation zone is most vulnerable to infection by HPV and an area of great focus during colposcopic examination (**Fig. 2**).

Indications

The indications for performing LEEP (**Table 2**) are based on the 2019 American Society for Colposcopy and Cervical Pathology (ASCCP) Risk-Based Management Consensus Guidelines for Abnormal Cervical Cancer Screening Tests and Cancer Precursors.[24] Compared with prior guidelines, the 2019 guidelines focus on the individual risk of developing CIN 3 or worse disease and recommend more expedited treatment. LEEP is preferred over cryotherapy and other ablative procedures in patients with an irregular ectocervix, lesions larger than the cryoprobe used for

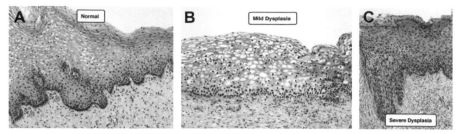

Fig. 1. Hematoxylin and eosin (H&E)-stained normal (*A*) tissue and tissue demonstrating cervical intraepithelial (CIN) of the cervix. CIN is classified from mild (*B*) to moderate to severe (*C*) (CINI, CIN II, CINIII). This classification is based on the appearance of nuclei, larger and darker in more severe forms of CIN, and the presence of basal cells in the upper part of the epithelium. Basal cells confined to the lower third indicate a low-grade lesion, whereas basal cells in the upper two-third indicate a high-grade lesion. (*Adapted from* Medical Cell Biology: A Collection of Resources for Cell Biology in Medical Education. http://medcell.med. yale.edu/histology/female_reproductive_system_lab/cervical_intraepithelial_neoplasia.php. Accessed January 28, 2021.)

cryotherapy or involving more than 3 quadrants, complex-appearing lesions with prominent abnormal vessels, and recurrent CIN after prior treatment.

Contraindications

- Known bleeding disorders
- Pregnancy
- Infectious or inflammatory processes present in the cervix at the time of evaluation.
- Patients diagnosed with lesions in the endocervical canal in whom LEEP would not be able to achieve clear margins or those with obvious cancer on visual or

Table 1
Bethesda Classification System for the reporting of cytologic and histologic abnormalities of the cervix

	Low-Grade Squamous Intraepithelial Lesion (LSIL)	High-Grade Squamous Intraepithelial Lesion (HSIL)	
Cytology		ASC-H	
Histology	CIN 1	CIN 2	CIN 3
Significance	• Mild dysplasia • Evidence of HPV infection • Confined to the basal 1/3 of the epithelium • Benign	• Moderate dysplasia • Confined to the basal 2/3 of the epithelium • Intermediate	• Severe dysplasia • Span more than 2/3 of the epithelium • Full-thickness neoplastic lesion • Also known as carcinoma in-situ
Likelihood of progressing to cancer	1%	5%	>12%

Abbreviation: ASC-H, Atypical squamous cells with high-grade squamous intraepithelial lesion.
Data from Refs.[21,23]

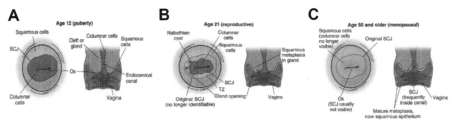

Fig. 2. Appearance of the cervix at puberty (*A*), during reproductive years (*B*), and once menopausal (*C*). The area most at risk in all age groups is the transformation zone (TZ), including the squamocolumnar junction (SCJ). Note how location varies with age. The SCJ and TZ are readily visible in younger women and may be quite large. The SCJ migrates inward with aging, and by menopause, it is usually within the canal and is not visible. The entire TZ must be sampled to maximize efficacy of the Pap smear. (*From* Newkirk GR. Chapter 120: Pap Smear and Related Techniques for Cervical Cancer Screening In: Fowler GC, ed. Pfenninger & Fowler's Procedures for Primary Care, 4th edition. Elsevier; 2020:814-824.)

Table 2 Indications for LEEP	
HSIL on cytology and HPV 16 positive	LEEP preferred[a]
HSIL on cytology and HPV 18 or other high risk positive	LEEP acceptable[a]
AGC (favor neoplasia) or AIS on cytology	LEEP preferred[a]
ASC-H on cytology and CIN 1 on colposcopy, age <25 y	LEEP preferred if ASC-H or HSIL present on follow-up cytology at 2 y
ASC-H on cytology and CIN 1 on colposcopy, age ≥25 y	LEEP preferred if ASC-H still present on follow-up cytology at 2 y or HSIL present on follow-up cytology at 1 or 2 y.
HSIL on cytology and CIN 1 on colposcopy	LEEP acceptable[b]
HSIL on cytology and unsatisfactory colposcopy	LEEP preferred[c]
CIN 2 or CIN 3 on colposcopy	LEEP preferred
CIN 2 or CIN 3 on endocervical sampling	LEEP preferred[c]

Abbreviations: ASC-H, Atypical squamous cells with high-grade squamous intraepithelial lesion; AIS, Adenocarcinoma In Situ; HSIL, high-grade squamous intraepithelial lesion.

[a] Colposcopy and LEEP can be performed on the same day, a technique commonly referred to as "see and treat."[5]

[b] If the patient chooses observation and HSIL persists on cytology at 1 y, LEEP is preferred.

[c] These patients should undergo LEEP conization, commonly referred to as "Top Hat LEEP".

Data from Perkins RB, Guido RS, Castle PE, et al. 2019 ASCCP risk-based management consensus guidelines for abnormal cervical cancer screening tests and cancer precursors. J Low Genit Tract Dis. 2020;24:102-131.

colposcopic examination. These patients should be referred for alternative surgical techniques.

PREPROCEDURAL PREPARATION
Equipment Needed

- Electrosurgical unit (ESU) with minimum 50-W output capability, patient grounding pad monitor, and isolated circuitry
- Nonconductive speculum (metal coated with nonconductive material or plastic) with smoke evacuator attachment
- Smoke evacuator with filter
- Colposcope
- Coated instruments including vaginal sidewall retractor, single-tooth tenaculum, ring forceps, endocervical speculum
- Loop electrodes (various sizes) and a ball electrode for fulguration
- Electrode handle
- Kevorkian endocervical curette
- Patient grounding pad
- 5% acetic acid
- Lugol's solution
- 1% to 2% lidocaine with 1:100,000 epinephrine
- 5 mL or 10 mL syringe with either a needle extender and 1.5-inch 25- to 27-gauge needle or a dental syringe with 25- to 27-gauge Potocky Needle
- Monsel's solution
- Vaginal packing
- Long needle holder and appropriate absorbable suture material (eg, Vicryl)

Patient Considerations

Patients should be counseled on the different treatment options, and informed consent should be obtained before starting the procedure. While evidence of benefit is lacking for the use of nonsteroidal anti-inflammatory drugs for pain control,[25] most providers still recommend that patients take 600 mg to 800 mg of ibuprofen before the procedure. Before starting the procedure, the ESU should be tested for proper function. The clinician should also verify that all needed equipment is available.

Procedural Approach

Initial equipment and patient preparation

1. With the patient on the examination table and in the lithotomy position, the grounding pad for the ESU is attached on the posterior thigh as close to the surgical site as possible.
2. A nonconductive speculum with the smoke evacuator attached is used to directly visualize the cervix. The cervix should be positioned as perpendicular to the performing provider as possible. A vaginal sidewall retractor can also be used if needed.
3. The cervix is examined with the colposcope to locate the transformation zone and to identify any unusual appearing areas. Acetic acid and/or Lugol's solution can be used to accentuate the appearance of abnormal cells.
4. The cervix is anesthetized using 1% or 2% lidocaine with epinephrine 1:100,000. An intracervical block is preferred; a paracervical block tends to be more painful.[25] Approximately 0.5 to 1 mL of lidocaine is injected just beneath (~2 mm) the surface of the cervix at the 12, 3, 6, and 9 o'clock positions. Additional injections can be performed for patients with a larger cervix.

Electrode Selection

When choosing an electrode, the provider should take into consideration the overall size of the disease, its location on the cervix and/or endocervical canal, and the potential for crypt involvement. The goal of treatment is to remove the entire lesion with at least a 2-mm margin while also sparing as much normal tissue as possible. Examples include

- For most patients, a round 2-cm-wide × 0.8-cm-deep loop will be sufficient to remove the entire lesion.
- For a smaller cervix (nulliparous patient, postmenopausal patient), a smaller loop such as 1.5-cm-wide × 0.7-cm-deep loop may be used.
- A 1-cm-wide × 1-cm-deep electrode can be used to remove the endocervical canal for "Top Hat" LEEP.

The settings for the ESU are generally provided by the manufacturer and can vary based on the size and type of electrode being used.

- Blended current offers both cutting and coagulation currents which allows for control of bleeding while leaving limited burn artifact on the obtained specimen.
- If using pure cutting current, a lower power setting should be used to avoid burn artifact.

Excision

Four types of excisional approaches have been described.[10,26–28] The excision can be performed under colposcopic or direct visualization depending on the preference and experience of the provider. One technique is to mark the targeted insertion and removal locations under colposcopy and then perform the full excision under direct visualization. A test pass can be performed to verify if the cutting path is free of obstruction.

1. Removal of ectocervical tissue with a single pass. The ESU should be activated just before touching the electrode to the tissue. The electrode is then inserted straight into the tissue and with a smooth motion drawn horizontally across the lesion, taking care to maintain constant depth, to the target removal site where it is then withdrawn. A 1- to 2-mm margin should be achieved on both sides of the lesion, and the entire transformation zone removed (**Fig. 3**). A vertical approach can be used; however, the specimen may need to be held up with a cotton swab to prevent it from falling over and impeding removal of the electrode. Care should be taken when removing the electrode to not contact any additional cervical or vaginal tissue. A cotton swab or wooden tongue depressor can be used to protect the surrounding tissue.
2. Removal of ectocervical tissue with multiple passes. Roughly 90% of lesions can be removed in a single pass.[5] When this is not possible, the general approach is to first remove as much from the center of the lesion, including the transformation zone, as possible. Repeat passes then can be taken to remove any additional remaining lesion from around the perimeter of the first pass (**Fig. 4**).
3. Excision of primarily endocervical CIN. Up to 86% of CIN 3 endocervical lesions are less than 10 mm in depth and can be treated with single-pass LEEP as described previously.[5] Deeper lesions are treated with LEEP conization (described in the following paragraph) or cylindrical needle excision. Needle excision uses a straight needle electrode to make circular cuts around the endocervix. Long forceps are used to help keep traction on the specimen until the appropriate depth is achieved. The cylindrical specimen is then cut at the apex with a scalpel. Needle excision may

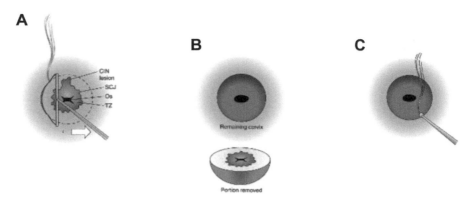

Fig. 3. (*A*) Standard loop electrosurgical excision procedure for cervical intraepithelial lesions that can be removed in a single pass (arrow indicates the direction of excision). (*B*) After painting the cervix with Lugol solution and injecting lidocaine, the clinician uses an ectocervical loop (2 cm wide and 0.8 cm deep) to resect the entire lesion. (*C*) The crater base is then coagulated using a 5-mm ball electrode followed by the application of Monsel's paste. (*From* Wright TC. Chapter 127: Loop electrosurgical excision procedure for treating cervical intraepithelial neoplasia. In: Fowler GC, ed. Pfenninger & Fowler's Procedures for Primary Care, 4th ed. Elsevier; 2020: 867-875.)

be better performed in an operating room[28] but can be carried out safely in the outpatient setting.[29]

4. Excision when there is both ectocervical and endocervical disease. Nearly 20% of all ectocervical CIN lesions will also extend into the endocervical canal, and thus, "Top Hat" LEEP is especially useful. The ectocervical component is typically excised first with a standard 2-cm × 0.8-cm loop electrode. Then, a 1-cm × 1-cm electrode is used to make a second pass over the endocervical canal to remove any remaining lesion. Care should be taken not to extend deeply into the endocervical canal. Alternatively, the smaller loop may be used first over the canal followed by the larger loop across the ectocervical portion of the lesion (**Fig. 5**).

Final Steps

1. The excised specimen(s) is removed with forceps, placed in an appropriate fixative solution, and sent for pathologic review. Some pathologists prefer the specimen to be tagged at a particular location with a small suture.
2. Carefully reinspect the cervix to ensure no residual abnormal tissue remains. If necessary, more acetic acid can be applied to aid in visualization of abnormal tissue. If there are remaining acetowhite changes—tissue that appears white after application of acetic acid—observed, additional excision should be done until all acetowhite areas are removed.
3. ECC is next performed to ensure no dysplasia is present above the excision.
4. Finally, fulguration with a ball electrode and/or Monsel's solution can be used for hemostasis. Heavier bleeding may require vaginal packing.

Postprocedural Care

Patients should be counseled to observe pelvic rest (ie, nothing per vagina) for 3 to 4 weeks. Most patients are completely healed by 21 days. At that point, follow-up in the office is recommended to review pathology, examine for healing, and recounsel on preventive measures such as HPV vaccination and tobacco cessation.

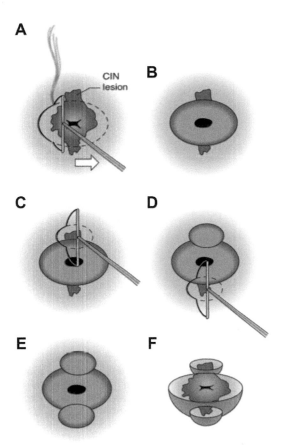

Fig. 4. (*A-B*) For lesions too large to be removed in a single pass, the clinician uses a 2.0-0.8cm loop electrode to resect the central portion of the lesion (arrow indicates direction of excision). (*C-E*) Remaining tissue is then resected with additional passes using the same electrode. (*F*) Tissue specimens are placed in the same bottle of formalin. (*From* Wright TC. Chapter 127: Loop electrosurgical excision procedure for treating cervical intraepithelial neoplasia. In: Fowler GC, ed. Pfenninger & Fowler's Procedures for Primary Care, 4th ed. Elsevier; 2020: 867-875.)

The 2019 ASCCP guidelines recommend HPV-based Pap testing at 6 months after the procedure. Any positive results (HPV or cytology) should be re-evaluated with colposcopy and managed accordingly. If testing remains negative, patients should be retested yearly for the first 3 years and then every 3 years for a minimum of 25 years after excision.[24]

Complications/Concerns

- Bleeding: The most common complication of LEEP is bleeding.
  - Heavy bleeding during the procedure is uncommon if the blended energy setting is used but can occur if the clinician cuts one of the cervical branches of the uterine arteries located at the 3 and 9 o'clock positions. Direct pressure and coagulation with the ball electrode can be used to achieve hemostasis. An injection of 1% to 2% lidocaine with epinephrine can also help control bleeding.

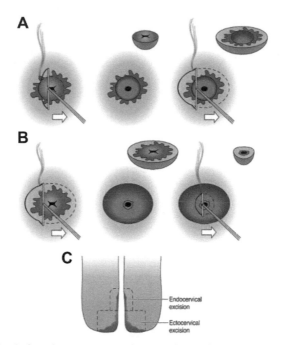

Fig. 5. Two methods for obtaining an endocervical sample with the loop electrosurgical excision procedure. (*A*) The clinician resects the endocervical portion of the lesion using a 1x1cm loop. A 2.0x0.8cm loop is then used to resect additional cervical intraepithelial neoplasia extending onto the portio (*arrow* indicates direction of excision). (*B*) In some cases it may be necessary to excise the ectocervical portion first. Excising to a depth greater than 1.5cm into the canal increases the chances of significant bleeding (*arrow* indicates direction of excision). (*C*) Longitudinal section showing the "top hat" procedure. (*From* Wright TC. Chapter 127: Loop electrosurgical excision procedure for treating cervical intraepithelial neoplasia. In: Fowler GC, ed. Pfenninger & Fowler's Procedures for Primary Care, 4th ed. Elsevier; 2020: 867-875.)

- ○ Postprocedural bleeding occurs in 4% to 6% of cases. Mild spotting can be seen during the first 1 to 2 weeks after the procedure and after initial intercourse. Heavier bleeding can often be treated in the office with Monsel's solution, vaginal packing, and/or cauterization; cervical sutures are rarely required. The risk of bleeding is greatest 6 to 10 days after the procedure.[26,27]
- Infections: Postprocedural infection after LEEP is rare and may be treated with either metronidazole or doxycycline.
- Cervical stenosis: Cervical stenosis complicates fewer than 1% of LEEP procedures.[6] Risk of cervical stenosis is higher in women who are amenorrheic, either directly postpartum or perimenopausal. Decreased estrogen levels can increase the risk of postprocedural cervical stenosis. At-risk patients can be pretreated with a combination oral contraceptive pill (OCP) for 3 to 4 cycles before, during, and after the procedure to reduce risk. For patients who are breastfeeding, vaginal estrogen cream can be used instead of OCPs. At-risk patients should be examined every 2 weeks for 6 to 8 weeks after the procedure to evaluate for cervical stenosis.[5]
- Cervical insufficiency and preterm delivery: The risk of adverse obstetric outcomes after excisional procedures such as CKC biopsy (cervical conization)

had been well established before the development of LEEP. Several systematic reviews have evaluated this risk in patients who have undergone LEEP and found a similar increased risk of preterm delivery, low birthweight, and premature rupture of membranes.[30,31] Based on these results, one can expect one excess preterm birth for every 18 LEEPs performed. Risk increases in those patients requiring multiple treatments. Studies comparing LEEP with CKC found the risk of preterm delivery was higher after CKC.[14]

SUMMARY

While the overall rates of cervical cancer in the US have decreased over recent years, the importance of surveillance and treatment was highlighted in the 2019 ASCCP guidelines which emphasize a risk-based approach and are more permissive of the use of LEEP for treatment of cervical dysplasia. When determining specific treatment options, providers must consider the patient's age, colposcopic findings, and desire for future pregnancy.

CLINICS CARE POINTS

- Offer LEEP to any patient with a high risk of CIN 3 based on initial cytology and HPV testing.
- Intracervical local anesthesia is more effective for pain control during LEEP than a paracervical block and is the recommended technique.
- When compared with blended cut energy, pure cut energy is easier to use, less likely to stall, and uses less power in turn reducing the risk of burn artifact but is less effective at hemostasis.
- If the electrode will not cut when touching the cervix, try wetting the tissue with acetic acid and ensure that the ESU is activated before touching the tissue with the electrode.
- Patients with hypoestrogenic states (eg, postpartum, perimenopausal) should be treated with a combination OCP or vaginal estrogen cream to reduce the risk of cervical stenosis.

DISCLOSURE

Dr. Ramirez is a certified Nexplanon Instructor.

REFERENCES

1. Siegel RL, Miller KD, Jemal A. Cancer statistics, 2020. CA Cancer J Clin 2020; 70:7.
2. Markowitz LE, Gee J, Chesson H, et al. Ten Years of Human Papillomavirus Vaccination in the United States. Acad Pediatr 2018;18(2S):S3–10.
3. Ferenczy A, Choukroun D, Arseneau J. Loop electrosurgical excision procedure for squamous intraepithelial lesions of the cervix: Advantages and potential pitfalls. Obstet Gynecol 1996;87(3):332–7.
4. Ferris DG, Hainer BL, Pfenninger JL, et al. Electrosurgical loop excision of the cervical transformation zone: The experience of family physicians. J Fam Pract 1995;41(4):337–44.
5. Cox JT, Ferris DG, Wright VC, et al. Management of lower genital tract neoplasia. In: Mayeaux EJ, Cox JT, editors. Modern colposcopy Textbook & Atlas. 3rd ed. Philadelphia: LWW; 2012. p. 637–47.

6. Wright TC. Loop electrosurgical excision procedure for treating cervical intraepithelial neoplasia. In: Fowler GC, editor. Pfenninger & Fowler's procedures for primary care. 4th ed. Philadelphia: Elsevier; 2020. p. 867–75.

7. Huang L-W, Huang J-L. A comparison between loop electrosurgical excision procedure and cold knife conization for the treatment of cervical dysplasia: residual disease in a subsequent hysterectomy specimen. Gynecol Oncol 1999;73:12–5.

8. Baggish MS, Barash F, Noel Y, et al. Comparison of thermal injury zone in loop electrical and laser excisional conization. Am J Obstet Gynecol 1992;166:545–8.

9. Wright TC, Richart RM, Ferenczy A, et al. Comparison of specimens removed by CO2 laser conization and loop electrosurgical procedures. Obstet Gynecol 1991; 79:147–53.

10. Darwish A, Gadallah H. One step management of cervical lesions. Int J Gynaecol Obstet 1998;61:261–7.

11. Simmons JR, Anderson L, Hernadez E, et al. Evaluating cervical neoplasia. LEEP as an alternative to cold knife conization. J Reprod Med 1998;43:1007–13.

12. Takac I, Gorisek B. Cold knife conization and loop excision for cervical intraepithelial neoplasia. Tumori 1999;85:243–6.

13. Giacalone PL, Laffargue F, Aligier N, et al. Randomized study comparing two techniques of conization: cold knife versus loop excision. Gynecol Oncol 1999; 75:356–60.

14. Santesso N, Mustafa RA, Wiercioch W, et al. Systematic reviews and meta-analyses of benefits and harms of cryotherapy, LEEP, and cold knife conization to treat cervical intraepithelial neoplasia. Int J Gynaecol Obstet 2016;132(3): 266–71.

15. National Program of Cancer Registries SEER*Stat Database: U.S. Cancer Statistics Incidence Analytic file 1998–2017. United States Department of Health and Human Services, Centers for Disease Control and Prevention. Released June 2020, based on the 2019 submission. Available at: https://www.cdc.gov/cancer/hpv/statistics/cases.htm. Accessed January 25, 2021.

16. U.S. Cancer Statistics Working Group. U.S. Cancer Statistics Data Visualizations Tool, based on 2019 submission data (1999-2017): U.S. Department of Health and Human Services, Centers for Disease Control and Prevention and National Cancer Institute. 2020. Available at: www.cdc.gov/cancer/dataviz. Accessed January 26, 2021.

17. McClung NM, Gargano JW, Park IU, et al. Estimated number of cases of high-grade cervical lesions diagnosed among women — United States, 2008 and 2016. MMWR Morb Mortal Wkly Rep 2019;68:337–43. Available at: https://doi.org/10.15585/mmwr.mm6815a1. Accessed January 26, 2021.

18. Del Priore G, Gudipudi DK, Montemarano N, et al. Oral diindolylmethane (DIM): pilot evaluation of a nonsurgical treatment for cervical dysplasia. Gynecol Oncol 2010;116(3):464–7.

19. Bogani G, Di Donato V, Sopracordevole F. Recurrence rate after loop electrosurgical excision procedure (LEEP) and laser conization: a 5-year follow-up study. Gynecol Oncol 2020;159(3):636–41.

20. Manos MM, Kinney WK, Hurley LB, et al. Identifying women with cervical neoplasia: using Human Papillomavirus DNA Testing for equivocal papanicolaou results. J Am Med Assoc 1999;281(17):1605–10.

21. Nayar R, Wilbur DC. The pap test and Bethesda 2014. J Lower Genital Tract Dis 2015;19(3):175–84.

22. Kim TJ, Kim HS, Park CT, et al. Clinical evaluation of follow-up methods and results of atypical glandular cells of undetermined significance (AGUS) detected on cervicovaginal Pap smears. Gynecol Oncol 1999;73:292–8.
23. Preinvasive lesions of the lower genital Tract. In: Hoffman BL, Schorge JO, Halvorson LM, et al. eds. Williams Gynecology, 4e. McGraw-Hill. Available at: http://accessmedicine.mhmedical.com/content.aspx?aid=1171532888. Accessed January 25, 2021.
24. Perkins RB, Guido RS, Castle PE, et al. 2019 ASCCP risk-based management consensus guidelines for abnormal cervical cancer screening tests and cancer precursors. J Low Genit Tract Dis 2020;24:102–31.
25. Gajjar K, Martin-Hirsch PPL, Bryant A, et al. Pain relief for women with cervical intraepithelial neoplasia undergoing colposcopy treatment. Cochrane Database Syst Rev 2016;(7). Art. No.: CD006120. Available at: https://www.cochranelibrary.com/cdsr/doi/10.1002/14651858.CD006120.pub4/full?highlightAbstract=leep. Accessed January 31, 2021.
26. Wright TC, Gagnon S, Richart RM, et al. Treatment of cervical intraepithelial neoplasia using the loop electrosurgical excision procedure. Obstet Gynecol 1992;79:173–8.
27. Prendiville W, Cullimore J, Norman S. Large loop excision of the transformation zone (LLETZ): a new method of management for women with intraepithelial neoplasia. Br J Obstet Gynecol 1989;96:1054–60.
28. Wright VC. Loop electrosurgical procedures for treatment of cervical intraepithelial neoplasia: principles and results. In: Wright VC, Lickrish GM, Shier RM, editors. Basic and Advanced colposcopy—Part Two: a Practical Handbook for treatment. 2nd ed. Houston, TX: Biomedical Communications; 1995. 20/1–20/31.
29. Sadek AL. Needle excision of the transformation zone: a new method for treatment of cervical intraepithelial neoplasia. Am J Obstet Gynecol 2000;182:866–71.
30. Crane JM. Pregnancy outcome after loop electrosurgical excision procedure: a systematic review. Obstet Gynecol 2003;102(5, pt 1):1058–62.
31. Kyrgiou M, Koliopoulos G, Martin-Hirsch P, et al. Obstetrical outcomes after conservative treatment for intraepithelial or early invasive cervical lesions: systematic review and meta-analysis. Lancet 2006;367:489–98.

Neonatal Circumcision

Matthew Zeitler, MD*, Brian Rayala, MD

KEYWORDS

- Newborn/neonatal • Circumcision • Gomco • Mogen • Plastibell

KEY POINTS

- Neonatal male circumcision, removal of the foreskin covering the glans penis, is one of the most common elective surgical procedures performed in the United States and globally.
- Circumcision remains controversial, but unbiased access is endorsed by major medical societies and organizations.
- Proposed benefits include lower rates of urinary tract infection, penile cancer, phimosis, penile dermatoses, HIV, and other sexually transmitted infections. More data are needed on the preventive and medical value in the United States.
- Three techniques, the Gomco, Plastibell, and Mogen, are equally safe and effective when used by a trained clinician.
- Complications are rare overall and include bleeding, injury, infection, and, even rarer, late complications.

INTRODUCTION/HISTORY/DEFINITIONS/BACKGROUND

Neonatal male circumcision is a common elective surgical procedure for the removal of the prepuce or foreskin covering the glans penis. Circumcision is centuries old and one of the most common procedures performed in the world. It is done for a variety of medical, cultural, and religious purposes. Neonatal circumcision is most often performed in the first days of life and can be accomplished through a variety of safe techniques. Newborn circumcision remains a controversial procedure with potential prospective medical benefits as well as disadvantages, risks, and ethical considerations. The American Academy of Pediatrics (AAP), the American College of Obstetricians and Gynecologists, the Centers for Disease Control and Prevention, the World Health Organization (WHO), and the American Academy of Family Physicians recognize the potential health benefits of newborn male circumcision and recommend access for families who choose this procedure. However, they do not universally recommend the procedure.[1–4] Despite its long history, common use globally, and varied organizational recommendations for unbiased access, some controversy remains about the procedure's medical and social value.[5]

Department of Family Medicine, University of North Carolina, 590 Manning Drive, Chapel Hill, NC 27599-7595, USA
* Corresponding author.
E-mail address: mzeitler@med.unc.edu

Prim Care Clin Office Pract 48 (2021) 597–611
https://doi.org/10.1016/j.pop.2021.08.002
0095-4543/21/© 2021 Elsevier Inc. All rights reserved.

NATURE OF THE PROBLEM/DIAGNOSIS

Approximately 1 in 3 boys and men worldwide are circumcised.[3] In the United States, most male infants are circumcised for nonreligious reasons. The rate of neonatal circumcision varies widely by region, race, socioeconomic status, and insurance coverage. The overall prevalence is estimated to be approximately 80% for boys and men aged 14 to 59 years, with most of these procedures performed in newborns. Rates have been falling over the last 2 decades.[6] Between 2003 and 2016, approximately 4.4 million boys underwent neonatal circumcision.[7] US physician perspectives on circumcision also fluctuate. In 2008, only about one-third of physicians surveyed thought that the benefits of male circumcision outweighed the risks and recommended the procedure.[8]

Circumcision rates outside of the United States vary, with an estimated global prevalence of 37% to 39%.[9] According to the WHO, there are several advantages of circumcising male infants in the newborn period, including a lower risk of complications, faster healing, and lower cost. The frequency of adverse events is 0.4% for circumcision during the first year of life, but this number increases 10 to 20 times in older boys and men.[3,4,10] Neonatal circumcision is performed by family physicians, pediatricians, obstetricians, urologists, and general surgeons.

ANATOMY

Knowledge of surgical anatomy is critical to ensure a safe, effective, and efficient circumcision. Male external genitalia begins development at 7 weeks' gestation. The penis develops as a tricylinder structure with bilateral dorsal corpora cavernosa (erectile bodies) and ventral midline corpus spongiosum, which surrounds the urethra. The penis is divided into the proximal base, middle shaft, and distal glans. The corona of the glans and coronal sulcus anatomically differentiate the glans penis from the penile shaft (**Fig. 1**).

The foreskin begins development at 12 weeks of gestation as an epithelial fold at the base of the penis that becomes a 5-layered prepuce covering the entire glans by 18 to 20 weeks. Development of the foreskin coincides with growth of the penis. The inner mucosal layer of the prepuce is adherent to the glans. Circumcision removes the inner and outer layers of the prepuce as well as the intervening dartos muscle.[11]

The penile skin and prepuce are innervated by the dorsal nerve, a terminal branch of the pudendal nerve. The main blood supply is the internal pudendal artery, whereas venous drainage occurs through the deep dorsal vein. The cavernosal, dorsal, and bulbourethral arteries and veins are branches of these 2 main blood vessels. In newborns, preputial adhesion between the glans and foreskin is normal, which creates a physiologic phimosis, or inability of the foreskin to retract over the glans penis. In natural progression of uncircumcised penile growth, the foreskin becomes more retractable over time with epithelial shedding (smegma) and intermittent erections causing progressive lysis of these adhesions.[4]

PREOPERATIVE/PREPROCEDURE PLANNING

Newborn circumcision may occur in the inpatient setting following in-hospital birth or outpatient setting upon discharge. A preoperative consultation with the family should be conducted, preferably in person. If in-person consultation is not possible, then virtual consultation by telephone, video, or electronic communication is an acceptable alternative.[2]

Physicians should accurately and impartially present information about potential benefits and risks of circumcision, and parents' decisions regarding the procedure

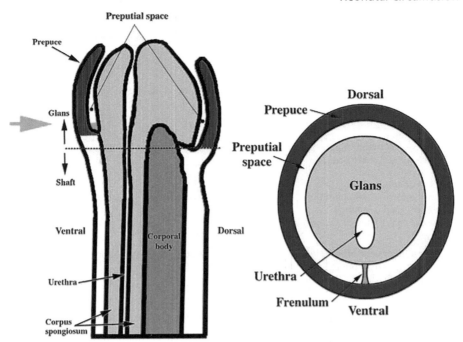

Fig. 1. Anatomy of the penis and prepuce. (*From* Cunha GR, Sinclair A, Cao M, Baskin LS. Development of the human prepuce and its innervation. Differentiation. 2020 Jan-Feb;111:22-40.)

should be respected. The decision to circumcise a newborn male infant is affected by parents' values and beliefs.[1,2] Furthermore, physicians should ensure that parents understand that circumcision is an elective procedure. Ideally, parents should receive this information in the preconception period or during pregnancy and determine what is in the best interest of their child. It is important to recognize that there can be intraparental disagreement about the decision to circumcise the infant. This disagreement should be resolved by the couple before proceeding, and circumcision should be delayed if no resolution is reached.[1,4,12–14] Another important ethical consideration is the child patient's inability to independently consent for permanent surgical alteration of his genitals, a psychosexually and functionally significant part of the body. Ethical opponents of circumcision argue that this procedure removes anatomically normal tissue with no urgent medical need and without patient consent.[15,16] Parents may consider deferring circumcision until their son reaches an age where he can make an informed decision. They should be counseled that circumcision performed in older children and adults has greater risks and costs, more postoperative discomfort, and a longer recovery period than newborn circumcision.[17] This situation is further complicated by the fact that there are social, cultural, religious, and familial benefits and harms that should be considered as well.[1] Medical professional societies in the United States ultimately support the principle that the decision to circumcise and its timing should be left up to parents after counseling. Written informed parental consent should be obtained before surgery.[1,2,13,18]

CONTRAINDICATIONS

There are anatomic and medical contraindications to newborn circumcision summarized in **Box 1**. Newborns with abnormal genitourinary anatomy should be referred to a pediatric urologist. In some cases, an anatomic abnormality may not be recognized

---

Box 1
Contraindications to circumcision

Circumcision contraindications

Anatomic
  Chordee: Congenital abnormality of penile curvature
  Concealed or buried penis or large suprapubic fat pad
  Micropenis
  Congenital megaprepuce: Significant redundancy of the inner preputial skin over a penis with normal shaft and glans
  Epispadias
  Hypospadias
  Penile torsion (median raphe 90° or greater about the shaft of the penis)
  Penoscrotal webbing
  Significant penile or foreskin edema

Medical
  Unstable or premature infant admitted to the neonatal intensive care unit
  Age less than 12 hours
  Bleeding diathesis
  Current illness
  Jaundice
  Lack of vitamin K administration or parental refusal is a relative contraindication

Data from Prabhakaran S, Ljuhar D, Coleman R, Nataraja RM. Circumcision in the pediatric patient: A review of indications, technique and complications. J Paediatr Child Health. 2018 Dec;54(12):1299-1307.

---

until the procedure is in progress. In newborns with hypospadias and an intact prepuce, circumcision can be safely completed. Aborting the procedure in this circumstance may expose the child to additional procedures under general anesthesia.[19] If other abnormalities are encountered intraoperatively, a urologic surgeon should be consulted.

Premature infants should have circumcision postponed until they are otherwise healthy and preparing for discharge.

POTENTIAL BENEFITS OF CIRCUMCISION TO DISCUSS WITH PARENTS

Approximately half of uncircumcised men and boys will experience an adverse foreskin-related medical condition over their lifetime.[20] Circumcision has been associated with several potential medical benefits, including lower rates of urinary tract infection (UTI), penile cancer, phimosis, penile dermatoses, HIV, and other sexually transmitted infections (STI).[21]

The evidence for potential benefit of circumcision is strongest for the prevention of UTI in male newborns during the first several months of life. The number needed to treat (NNT) to prevent 1 newborn male UTI is approximately 111 to 140 and to prevent 1 hospitalization for complicated UTI is 195.[18,22] UTI is uncommon in boys and men at any age, with higher prevalence in uncircumcised boys and men, particularly during infancy.[22,23] In most cases, UTI can be treated in the outpatient setting without sequelae. However, UTI can result in complicated illness, such as pyelonephritis, requiring hospitalization and, rarely, sepsis or death. In infants with congenital uropathy, UTI can have serious consequences, and circumcision may have greater benefit.[24,25] Over a man's lifetime, lack of circumcision may confer a risk of UTI exceeding 20%.[26]

Circumcision may prevent penile cancer, but this is a rare disease (0.6/100,000), and the NNT is approximately 300,000.[18,27] Penile hygiene may be a confounding factor in data surrounding penile cancer reduction with circumcision; hygiene practices and access may change based on geographic location and circumstance.[27] In addition, approximately 30% of penile cancers is caused by human papilloma virus (HPV) and may be prevented by HPV immunization, which may diminish the preventive value of circumcision for penile malignancy.[16,18]

There is an inverse association between male circumcision and penile HPV infection, which confers a reduced risk of HPV transmission and subsequent cervical cancer to female partners, particularly among men with a history of multiple sexual partners. More studies are needed to adequately assess the effect of circumcision on the acquisition and clearance of HPV infections and transmission to partners.[28,29] Widespread HPV immunization may reduce the primary preventive value of circumcision for HPV transmission and cervical cancer.

There is also evidence that circumcision can prevent some other STIs, including HIV, HPV, HSV-2, and chancroid (*Haemophilus ducreyi*).[28,30–37] Most of the evidence for STI prevention comes from studies of voluntary adult circumcision in Africa and may not be generalizable to neonatal circumcision in the United States. The protective effects of circumcision on HIV acquisition are most clear for heterosexual men, with no data showing protective benefit for female partners and a paucity of data among the men who have sex with men population.[32–37] Data are also conflicting on circumcision affecting incidence of syphilis, perhaps because of low overall prevalence among study populations.[30,31] Circumcision does not protect against gonorrhea, chlamydia trachomatis, or trichomonas infections.[38] Circumcision should not be offered as the only strategy for HIV and other STI reduction and prevention; other methods of risk reduction, including safe sexual practices and barrier methods, should be emphasized.[2]

Finally, circumcision may prevent penile dermatoses, such as phimosis, paraphimosis, and balanoposthitis, but data are limited. These conditions can often be treated medically, and there is diminished preventive value with appropriate penile care and hygiene among uncircumcised boys and men.[4,16,25]

Before performing circumcision, a physical examination should be performed to evaluate anatomy and exclude congenital anomalies and procedural contraindications.

PREPARATION AND PATIENT POSITIONING

Before performing circumcision, the clinician should confirm that the patient has voided at least once since birth and received vitamin K, consistent with recommendations from the AAP.[1,39] In addition, routine patient safety protocols should be followed, such as confirming correct patient identity. Many institutions use a standardized circumcision kit, which contains the following materials and instruments:

- Restraint with padded leg straps for patient immobilization and support (infant holder with fastener straps)
- Local anesthetic and alcohol preparation pad
- Antiseptic agent: betadine or chlorhexidine
- Fenestrated drape and/or sterile towels
- Hemostats, straight and or blunt-edge scissors, blunt probe, safety pins
- Circumcision device (Gomco, Mogen, Plastibell) with appropriate sizes
- Hemostatic agents: Gauze, fine absorbable sutures, compressive dressing, aluminum chloride, silver nitrate, thrombin, or other hemostatic agents, such as Gelfoam or Surgicel
- Sucrose 24% on gloved finger or pacifier

- Postcircumcision dressing: Antibiotic ointment, petrolatum gauze, compressive dressing

Once a timeout has been performed and patient identity verified, the infant should be restrained. The penis should be inspected for abnormalities and normal position of the urethral meatus, median raphe, and scrotum. The penis and scrotum can be cleansed before or after local anesthesia administration with antiseptic solution. The remainder of the procedure should be performed using sterile technique. If antiseptic is not applied before anesthetic infiltration, an alcohol swab should be used to clean the injection site or sites for nerve blockade.

Anesthesia Approaches

Anesthesia should be administered to all newborns undergoing circumcision, regardless of technique.[1,2]

Application of topical lidocaine, prilocaine, or topical eutectic mixture of local anesthetic cream reduces the pain of the anesthetic injection and procedure when applied 30 to 60 minutes before the procedure. Alone, it is inferior to local anesthetic nerve blocks.[40–43]

A nerve block should be performed approximately 5 minutes before the procedure using 1% lidocaine with or without epinephrine. Classical teaching suggests avoiding epinephrine in anatomy perfused by terminal vessels. However, newer data in children 3 years and older and adults suggest that supplementing local anesthetic with epinephrine in penis operations has advantages, including lower complication rates, improved view of the operating field, and an extended effect of anesthetic with prolonged reduction in pain.[44] The objective is to anesthetize the 2 branches of the dorsal nerve that innervate the penis and foreskin. Two approaches are equally effective: the dorsal nerve block and the ring block.

For the dorsal penile nerve block, 0.2 to 0.4 mL of lidocaine is injected on either side of the base of the penis at 10 o'clock and 2 o'clock. This can be accomplished with 2 separate injections or 1 midline injection, with advancement of the needle laterally to inject medication at the correct positions. The clinician must take care to avoid the midline vasculature.

The ring block method requires a 0.8-mL injection circumferentially around the base of the penis. Lidocaine 0.4 mL is injected subcutaneously at the base of the penis transversely across the dorsal surface, and then the needle is introduced at the ventral base of the penis and advanced laterally to each side until anesthetic is infiltrated circumferentially. The ring block or dorsal penile nerve block is more effective than topical lidocaine/prilocaine alone.

Sucrose solution on a gloved finger or pacifier is an additional analgesic option. Recent randomized controlled trials comparing topical anesthetics alone with combination analgesics (topical, nerve block, sucrose) showed that combination analgesics, especially topical anesthetic plus sucrose plus ring block, are more effective.[4,40,42,43,45]

Injection that is too superficial can cause anesthetic to track along the penile shaft, which can distort the anatomy and complicate the circumcision. Alternatively, too deep an injection can cause vascular damage and lead to hematoma, penile distortion, and bleeding. Intravascular injection of local anesthetic should be avoided.

PROCEDURAL APPROACH

The 3 most common and equally effective techniques for circumcision use the Gomco clamp (**Fig. 2**), the Plastibell device (**Fig. 3**), and the Mogen clamp. Given equal

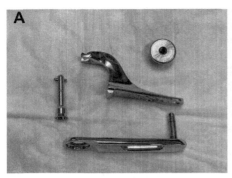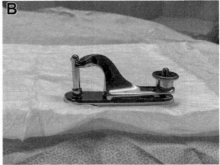

Fig. 2. Gomco clamp: (*A*) parts from left to right: bell, base plate, yoke, nut; (*B*) assembled.

efficacy, device choice should be guided by operator experience and comfort level. The Mogen and Gomco clamps protect the glans during foreskin excision, and the Plastibell device induces tissue necrosis, causing the foreskin to slough off along with the plastic shield within a week.[1,3,4,25,46–49] One randomized trial suggested that procedures using the Mogen clamp produce less pain than those using the Gomco clamp by physiologic measures (vital signs and salivary cortisol) but not clinical pain scores.[50] Use of the Gomco and Plastibell devices requires more training, takes longer to perform, and is associated with more bleeding and complications.[4,47,48,51]

The initial steps of the procedure are the same for all 3 devices[51]:

- Grasp the foreskin at the 3 and 9 o'clock or 10 and 2 o'clock positions with 2 hemostats.
- With gentle traction on the 2 hemostats, pass a straight clamp/hemostat into the preputial orifice, tenting dorsally to avoid meatal trauma, and sweep from side to side across the glans to break up adhesions. Care should be taken to avoid the ventral frenulum. Open the clamp and retract to gently stretch the preputial opening. Do not blindly reclose the clamp inside the foreskin. Care should also be taken not to accidently dissect the foreskin layers during this step and create a false lumen between tissue planes.
- With gentle traction on the hemostats, a straight clamp is placed and clamped in the midline of the dorsal foreskin to create an area of avascularity. The clamp

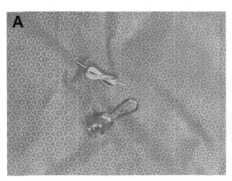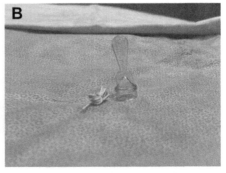

Fig. 3. Plastibell device.

should be kept in place for at least 30 seconds to devitalize the clamped foreskin. Straight or blunt tip scissors are then used to cut a dorsal slit, again taking care to tent the foreskin dorsally to ensure that the tip of 1 side of the scissors is visualized under the foreskin.

- To prevent separation of the preputial layers and proximal displacement of the internal layer, some operators suture the apex with 4-0 silk suture, leaving the length of suture on a hemostat.[52]
- Fully retract the foreskin; completely lyse any adhesions with a blunt probe or gauze, and clearly visualize the entire coronal sulcus.
- Of note, the dorsal slit and foreskin retraction are not required for the Mogen technique but can be used.

The photograph series in **Fig. 4** demonstrates these initial steps.

Method 1: Gomco Technique

The Gomco clamp device is made up of multiple parts (the bell, base plate, yoke, and nut) that result in a crushed tissue edge for hemostatic excision (**Fig. 2**).[4,25,47–49,51,53,54] The foreskin is removed with a scalpel during the procedure. The bell protects the glans and urethra from intraoperative injury. The Gomco bell ranges from 1.1 to 1.6 cm in diameter. Choice of device size depends on the diameter of the glans. The most commonly used size is 1.3 cm.[4,51,53]

- In the Gomco technique, the dorsal slit is made with blunt-edge scissors one-third to two-thirds the distance from the coronal margin (not closer than 1 cm to the coronal sulcus in the foreskin), and the foreskin is retracted to expose the glans.
- The Gomco bell is placed under the foreskin and over the glans, and the foreskin is pulled over the bell using the hemostats placed at the start of the procedure.
- A hemostat or a small safety pin is used to bring the edges of the dorsal incision together over the flare or shaft of the bell before the base plate is applied.
- The hemostats at the 10 and 2 o'clock positions are removed.
- The foreskin is gently pulled through the hole in the base plate if safety pinned or regrasped with another hemostat at 12 o'clock through the hole above the base plate, and the base plate is placed over the bell.
- The lip of the bell should align perfectly into the base plate without any gaps.
- The apex of the dorsal slit should be visible above the base plate.
- The yoke of the top plate (rocker arm) is attached to the arms of the bell.
- The other end of the top plate is tightened to the base plate with the nut and left in place for 5 minutes. The 5-minute time requirement is by procedural convention,

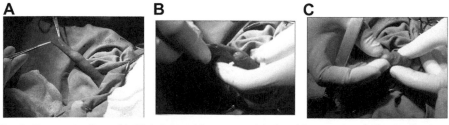

A   **B**   **C**

Fig. 4. Demonstration of Initial circumcision steps with foreskin grasping, lysis of adhesions, dorsal slit, and foreskin retraction to the coronal sulcus. (*From* Abdulwahab-Ahmed A, Mungadi IA. Techniques of male circumcision. J Surg Tech Case Rep. 2013 Jan;5(1):1–7.)

to allow sufficient tissue devitalization; however, there is no trial evidence to support the specific time duration.

- During this time, excess foreskin is excised with a scalpel flush against the base plate.
- After 5 minutes, the nut is loosened and the clamp disassembled. Gauze or a blunt probe is used to gently push the crushed foreskin off the bell (**Fig. 5**).

A video demonstrating a circumcision using the Gomco clamp is accessible at https://vimeo.com/74547358.

Method 2: Plastibell

The Plastibell device is a plastic bell with a groove on the outside that fits over the glans to protect it during the procedure (see **Fig. 3**).[4,25,47,48,51,52,54,55] A string is tied around the bell and is tightened in the groove to induce preputial necrosis. All devitalized foreskin distal to the ligature will necrose and fall away within 7 to 10 days with the plastic bell.[47] Using the protective bell, risk of injury to the glans or urethral meatus is minimal.

- In the Plastibell method, the dorsal slit is made identically to the Gomco procedure.
- Once the glans is freed, it should be calibrated with an appropriately sized Plastibell device, between 1.2 and 1.7 cm. The most common size is 1.3 cm.
- The Plastibell is placed under the foreskin and over the glans.
- Then the foreskin is pulled over the Plastibell with a hemostat and stabilized by clamping it to the handle of the Plastibell using a hemostat or safety pin.
- A second hemostat may be used to control the Plastibell by clamping it across the stem.
- Position the Plastibell so that the grooved ring is below the apex of the dorsal slit.
- The Plastibell is secured in place by tying a string around the groove on the bell, typically with a square knot, and the hemostats are removed.
- Excess foreskin past the outer edge is removed with a scalpel, and the handle is broken off, leaving the ring in place.
- The foreskin should be cut circumferentially approximately 2 mm distal to the string ligature using a scissors or a scalpel (**Fig. 6**).

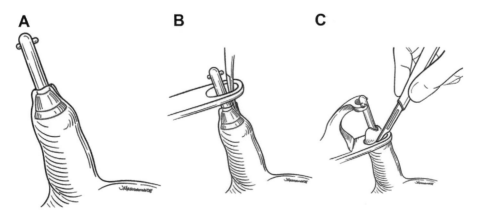

A   **B**   **C**

Fig. 5. Applying the Gomco clamp. (*From* Featherson, DO JS. Circumcision (procedure) [Internet]. Essential Evidence. 2019 [cited 2021 Jan 28]. Available at: https://www. essentialevidenceplus.com/content/eee/604.)

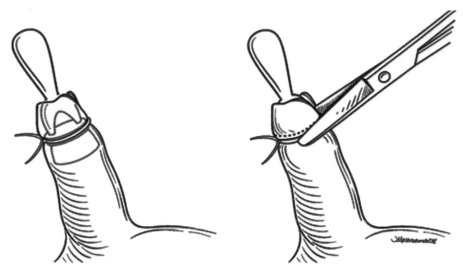

Fig. 6. Applying the Plastibell and removing distal foreskin. (*From* Featherson, DO JS. Circumcision (procedure) [Internet]. Essential Evidence. 2019 [cited 2021 Jan 28]. Available at: https://www.essentialevidenceplus.com/content/eee/604.)

- The ring and remaining necrotic preputial tissue will fall off within a week.

Method 3: Mogen[4,25,47,48,50,51,54]

- In the Mogen method, a dorsal slit is not necessary unless needed to fully retract the foreskin.
- Once coronal adhesions have been lysed, the glans is pushed downward.
- The foreskin, held with hemostats at 9 and 3 o'clock or 10 and 2 o'clock, is slid between the narrowly opened Mogen clamp to an approximate depth of 5 mm distal to the corona of the glans.
- Some operators will apply a dorsal hemostat at 12 o'clock (similar to the dorsal slit) or regrasp the edges of the dorsal slit (if performed) to retract the prepuce for clamp placement.
- The clamp is applied with the concave surface facing downward after ensuring that the glans is not caught in the clamp (**Fig. 7**).
- The clamp is closed and left in place for 60 to 90 seconds by convention.
- Excess foreskin is removed with a scalpel, and then the clamp is removed.

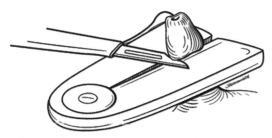

Fig. 7. The Mogen technique. (*From* Featherson, DO JS. Circumcision (procedure) [Internet]. Essential Evidence. 2019 [cited 2021 Jan 28]. Available from: https://www.essentialevidenceplus.com/content/eee/604.)

- A blunt probe or gauze is then used to gently separate the foreskin, pushing it down below the corona, fully exposing the glans.

A video demonstrating a circumcision using a Mogen clamp is available at https://med.stanford.edu/newborns/professional-education/circumcision/mogen-clamp-technique.html.

Mogen clamp circumcision can be completed in less than 5 minutes, whereas the Gomco clamp or Plastibell method can take up to 10 minutes. In general, the procedure time is inversely related to operator experience.[4]

COMPLICATIONS/OUTCOMES

Circumcision can result in immediate and later complications. The overall rate of post-procedural complications is estimated to be 2 to 6/1000. Acute complications include bleeding (0.8–1.8/1000), injury to the penis, including meatal trauma, glans injury, or rare penile amputation (0.4/1000), infection (0.6/1000), and unsatisfactory cosmesis, which is poorly defined. Minor bleeding is the most common early complication. Infants who are vitamin K deficient may have prolonged bleeding, and lack of vitamin K administration and parental refusal of vitamin K administration at birth are relative contraindications to the procedure. Postprocedure bleeding can occur for up to 8 weeks.[1,4,14,25,39,54,56–59]

Late complications are relatively rare and include incomplete circumcision, excessive skin removal, adhesions, meatal stenosis, phimosis, epidermal inclusion cysts, skin bridges, and abnormal scarring (including circumferential cicatrix). Rates of these late complications are not well defined. Patients with late complications should be referred to a pediatric urologist. Meatal stenosis can usually prevented by advising parents to apply petrolatum jelly liberally to the glans postprocedure.[4,20,25,46,54,56–58]

Wide-ranging evidence from surveys, physiologic measurements, and the anatomic location of penile sensory receptors responsible for sexual sensation consistently suggests that circumcision has no detrimental effect on sexual function, sensitivity, or satisfaction.[20,60]

There is also no evidence of an association between neonatal circumcision and breastfeeding initiation or outcomes.[61]

MANAGEMENT

If bleeding occurs intraoperatively or postoperatively, electrocautery should never be used in conjunction with metal instruments, as devastating penile loss can occur. Bleeding most commonly results from disruption of the frenular vessels, premature removal of clamps, mismatched Gomco bell and plate, or too loose a tie on the Plastibell string. Direct pressure should be applied immediately, which will stop most bleeding. If hemostasis is not achieved with direct pressure, a compressive wrap (eg, Coban) or hemostatic agents (eg, thrombin, Gelfoam, Surgicel, silver nitrate, or aluminum chloride) can be applied. Excessive bleeding, particularly from a visualized blood vessel, may require suturing and urology consultation. Infrequent wound infections typically resolve with topical antibiotic therapy and wound care. Rarely, systemic antibiotics, hospitalization, or surgical intervention is necessary. If injury occurs during the procedure, hemostasis should be attempted and urology consulted immediately.[4,25,54,59]

RECOVERY AND REHABILITATION (INCLUDING POSTPROCEDURE CARE)

There are no formal data to guide postcircumcision care. Choice of postprocedural dressing or topical agent is clinician dependent. Typically, a barrier cream, such as petrolatum jelly and gauze (eg, Xeroform), is applied to reduce the risk of penile adhesions and meatal stenosis.[62] This also prevents the diaper from sticking to the wound during the healing period, and causing pain. The newborn can be discharged from the hospital or clinic after 30 to 60 minutes of observation to ensure no excessive bleeding; it is not necessary to wait until a postprocedure void.

A skin barrier, such as petrolatum jelly, is recommended until the skin edge has fully healed, generally by 2 weeks. The shaft skin should not be forcibly retracted. Gentle retraction of the skin to visualize the incision and applying ointment may help reduce the rate of penile adhesions requiring revision. Written information describing postcircumcision care should be provided.

CLINICS CARE POINTS

- Parents should be offered newborn circumcision in a nonbiased conversation regarding potential risks, benefits, and ethical considerations.
- Local anesthesia should be provided during newborn circumcision using a dorsal nerve or ring block, alone or in combination with topical anesthetic agents and/or oral sucrose.
- Thorough lysis of adhesions between the glans and the foreskin facilitates the procedure.
- Use caution when manipulating the vascular penile frenulum.
- The Mogen clamp, the Gomco clamp, and the Plastibell device are all appropriate for newborn circumcision in trained hands.
- Infants with abnormal genitourinary anatomy should be referred to a pediatric urologist.

DISCLOSURE

The authors have nothing to disclose.

REFERENCES

1. American Academy of Pediatrics Task Force on Circumcision. Male circumcision. Pediatrics 2012;130(3):e756–85.
2. Circumcision - American Urological Association [Internet]. Available at: https://www.auanet.org/guidelines/circumcision. Accessed January 20, 2021.
3. Weiss. Neonatal and child male circumcision: a global review. UNAIDS; 2010. ISBN 978 92 9 173855 7.
4. Omole F, Smith W, Carter-Wicker K. Newborn circumcision techniques. Am Fam Physician 2020;101(11):680–5.
5. Piontek EA, Albani JM. Male circumcision: the clinical implications are more than skin deep. Mo Med 2019;116(1):35–7.
6. Morris BJ, Bailis SA, Wiswell TE. Circumcision rates in the United States: rising or falling? What effect might the new affirmative pediatric policy statement have? Mayo Clin Proc 2014;89(5):677–86.
7. Jacobson DL, Balmert LC, Holl JL, et al. Nationwide circumcision trends: 2003 to 2016. J Urol 2021;205(1):257–63.
8. Matar L, Zhu J, Chen RT, et al. Medical risks and benefits of newborn male circumcision in the United States: physician perspectives. J Int Assoc Provid AIDS Care 2015;14(1):33–9.
9. Morris BJ, Wamai RG, Henebeng EB, et al. Estimation of country-specific and global prevalence of male circumcision. Popul Health Metr 2016;14:4.

10. El Bcheraoui C, Zhang X, Cooper CS, et al. Rates of adverse events associated with male circumcision in U.S. medical settings, 2001 to 2010. JAMA Pediatr 2014;168(7):625–34.

11. Cold CJ, Taylor JR. The prepuce. BJU Int 1999;83(Suppl 1):34–44.

12. US Department of Health and Human Services. Draft CDC recommendations for providers counseling male patients and parents regarding male circumcision and the prevention of HIV infection, STIs, and other health outcomes. CDC; 2014 - 0012.

13. American College of Obstetricians and Gynecologists. Committee on Obstetric Practice. ACOG committee opinion. Circumcision. Number 260, October 2001. Obstet Gynecol 2001;98(4):707–8.

14. Pinto K. Circumcision controversies. Pediatr Clin North Am 2012;59(4):977–86.

15. Myers A, Earp BD. What is the best age to circumcise? A medical and ethical analysis. Bioethics 2020;34(7):645–63.

16. Hay W. Low specificity limits use of test for spondylolysis in children and adolescents. Am Fam Physician 2021;103(2):68.

17. Morris BJ, Waskett JH, Banerjee J, et al. A "snip" in time: what is the best age to circumcise? BMC Pediatr 2012;12:20.

18. Neonatal circumcision [Internet]. Available at: https://www.aafp.org/about/policies/all/neonatal-circumcision.html. Accessed January 27, 2021.

19. Chalmers D, Wiedel CA, Siparsky GL, et al. Discovery of hypospadias during newborn circumcision should not preclude completion of the procedure. J Pediatr 2014;164(5):1171–4.e1.

20. Morris BJ, Kennedy SE, Wodak AD, et al. Early infant male circumcision: systematic review, risk-benefit analysis, and progress in policy. World J Clin Pediatr 2017;6(1):89–102.

21. Tobian AAR, Gray RH. The medical benefits of male circumcision. JAMA 2011;306(13):1479–80.

22. Singh-Grewal D, Macdessi J, Craig J. Circumcision for the prevention of urinary tract infection in boys: a systematic review of randomised trials and observational studies. Arch Dis Child 2005;90(8):853–8.

23. Shaikh N, Morone NE, Bost JE, et al. Prevalence of urinary tract infection in childhood: a meta-analysis. Pediatr Infect Dis J 2008;27(4):302–8.

24. Ellison JS, Dy GW, Fu BC, et al. Neonatal circumcision and urinary tract infections in infants with hydronephrosis. Pediatrics 2018;142(1).

25. Baskin LS. UNC chapel hill libraries [Internet]. UpToDate; 2020. Available at: https://www-uptodate-com.libproxy.lib.unc.edu/contents/neonatal-circumcision-risks-and-benefits?search=newborn%20circumcision&source=search_result&selectedTitle=2~97&usage_type=default&display_rank=2#references. Accessed January 22, 2021.

26. Morris BJ, Wiswell TE. Circumcision and lifetime risk of urinary tract infection: a systematic review and meta-analysis. J Urol 2013;189(6):2118–24.

27. Larke NL, Thomas SL, dos Santos Silva I, et al. Male circumcision and penile cancer: a systematic review and meta-analysis. Cancer Causes Control 2011;22(8):1097–110.

28. Albero G, Castellsagué X, Giuliano AR, et al. Male circumcision and genital human papillomavirus: a systematic review and meta-analysis. Sex Transm Dis 2012;39(2):104–13.

29. Castellsagué X, Bosch FX, Muñoz N, et al. Male circumcision, penile human papillomavirus infection, and cervical cancer in female partners. N Engl J Med 2002;346(15):1105–12.

30. Tobian AAR, Serwadda D, Quinn TC, et al. Male circumcision for the prevention of HSV-2 and HPV infections and syphilis. N Engl J Med 2009;360(13):1298–309.
31. Weiss HA, Thomas SL, Munabi SK, et al. Male circumcision and risk of syphilis, chancroid, and genital herpes: a systematic review and meta-analysis. Sex Transm Infect 2006;82(2):101–9 [discussion 110].
32. Millett GA, Flores SA, Marks G, et al. Circumcision status and risk of HIV and sexually transmitted infections among men who have sex with men: a meta-analysis. JAMA 2008;300(14):1674–84.
33. Bailey RC, Moses S, Parker CB, et al. Male circumcision for HIV prevention in young men in Kisumu, Kenya: a randomised controlled trial. Lancet 2007; 369(9562):643–56.
34. Wawer MJ, Makumbi F, Kigozi G, et al. Circumcision in HIV-infected men and its effect on HIV transmission to female partners in Rakai, Uganda: a randomised controlled trial. Lancet 2009;374(9685):229–37.
35. Warner L, Ghanem KG, Newman DR, et al. Male circumcision and risk of HIV infection among heterosexual African American men attending Baltimore sexually transmitted disease clinics. J Infect Dis 2009;199(1):59–65.
36. Gray RH, Kigozi G, Serwadda D, et al. Male circumcision for HIV prevention in men in Rakai, Uganda: a randomised trial. Lancet 2007;369(9562):657–66.
37. Auvert B, Taljaard D, Lagarde E, et al. Randomized, controlled intervention trial of male circumcision for reduction of HIV infection risk: the ANRS 1265 Trial. Plos Med 2005;2(11):e298.
38. Mehta SD, Moses S, Agot K, et al. Adult male circumcision does not reduce the risk of incident Neisseria gonorrhoeae, Chlamydia trachomatis, or Trichomonas vaginalis infection: results from a randomized, controlled trial in Kenya. J Infect Dis 2009;200(3):370–8.
39. Plank RM, Steinmetz T, Sokal DC, et al. Vitamin K deficiency bleeding and early infant male circumcision in Africa. Obstet Gynecol 2013;122(2 Pt 2):503–5.
40. Wang J, Zhao S, Luo L, et al. Dorsal penile nerve block versus eutectic mixture of local anesthetics cream for pain relief in infants during circumcision: a meta-analysis. PLoS One 2018;13(9):e0203439.
41. White MA, Maatman TJ. Comparative analysis of effectiveness of two local anesthetic techniques in men undergoing no-scalpel vasectomy. Urology 2007;70(6):1187–9.
42. Taddio A, Ohlsson A, Ohlsson K. WITHDRAWN: lidocaine-prilocaine cream for analgesia during circumcision in newborn boys. Cochrane Database Syst Rev 2015;(4):CD000496.
43. Rossi S, Buonocore G, Bellieni CV. Management of pain in newborn circumcision: a systematic review. Eur J Pediatr 2021;180(1):13–20.
44. Schnabl SM, Herrmann N, Wilder D, et al. Clinical results for use of local anesthesia with epinephrine in penile nerve block. J Dtsch Dermatol Ges 2014; 12(4):332–9.
45. Stevens B, Yamada J, Ohlsson A, et al. Sucrose for analgesia in newborn infants undergoing painful procedures. Cochrane Database Syst Rev 2016;7:CD001069.
46. Prabhakaran S, Ljuhar D, Coleman R, et al. Circumcision in the paediatric patient: a review of indications, technique and complications. J Paediatr Child Health 2018;54(12):1299–307.
47. Abdulwahab-Ahmed A, Mungadi IA. Techniques of male circumcision. J Surg Tech Case Rep 2013;5(1):1–7.

48. Morris JB, Eley C. Male circumcision: an appraisal of current instrumentation. In: Fazel R, editor. Biomedical engineering - from theory to applications. InTech; 2011. https://doi.org/10.5772/18543.

49. Bawazir OA, Banaja AM. Sutureless versus interrupted sutures techniques for neonatal circumcision; a randomized clinical trial. J Pediatr Urol 2020;16(4): 493.e1–6.

50. Sinkey RG, Eschenbacher MA, Walsh PM, et al. The GoMo study: a randomized clinical trial assessing neonatal pain with Gomco vs Mogen clamp circumcision. Am J Obstet Gynecol 2015;212(5):664–e1–8.

51. Holman JR, Lewis EL, Ringler RL. Neonatal circumcision techniques. Am Fam Physician 1995;52(2):519.

52. Mahomed A, Zaparackaite I, Adam S. Improving outcome from Plastibell circumcisions in infants. Int Braz J Urol 2009;35(3):310–3 [discussion 313].

53. Peleg D, Steiner A. The Gomco circumcision: common problems and solutions. Am Fam Physician 1998;58(4):891–8.

54. Featherson DO. Circumcision (procedure) [Internet]. Essential Evidence; 2019. Available at: https://www.essentialevidenceplus.com/content/eee/604. Accessed January 28, 2021.

55. Al-Marhoon MS, Jaboub SM. Plastibell circumcision: how safe is it?: experience at Sultan Qaboos University Hospital. Sultan Qaboos Univ Med J 2006;6(1): 17–20.

56. Srinivasan M, Hamvas C, Coplen D. Rates of complications after newborn circumcision in a well-baby nursery, special care nursery, and neonatal intensive care unit. Clin Pediatr (Phila) 2015;54(12):1185–91.

57. Weiss HA, Larke N, Halperin D, et al. Complications of circumcision in male neonates, infants and children: a systematic review. BMC Urol 2010;10:2.

58. Earp BD. Do the benefits of male circumcision outweigh the risks? A critique of the proposed CDC guidelines. Front Pediatr 2015;3:18.

59. Heras A, Vallejo V, Pineda MI, et al. Immediate complications of elective newborn circumcision. Hosp Pediatr 2018;8(10):615–9.

60. Morris BJ, Krieger JN. Does male circumcision affect sexual function, sensitivity, or satisfaction?–A systematic review. J Sex Med 2013;10(11):2644–57.

61. Mondzelewski L, Gahagan S, Johnson C, et al. Timing of circumcision and breastfeeding initiation among newborn boys. Hosp Pediatr 2016;6(11):653–8.

62. Bazmamoun H, Ghorbanpour M, Mousavi-Bahar SH. Lubrication of circumcision site for prevention of meatal stenosis in children younger than 2 years old. Urol J 2008;5(4):233–6.

Outpatient Vasectomy
Safe, Reliable, and Cost-effective

Matthew Zeitler, MD*, Brian Rayala, MD

KEYWORDS

- Outpatient • Vasectomy • Contraception • Safety

KEY POINTS

- Vasectomy can be readily and safely performed in the outpatient setting.
- The preferred approach is the no-needle, no scalpel approach which utilizes jet injection anesthesia and one small scrotal incision with dissecting forceps to isolate the vas deferens (vas).
- The same midline scrotal incision is used to isolate both vas.
- The most effective method of vasectomy is vasal excision with end cauterization and fascial interposition of the prostatic end.
- Sterility must be confirmed by semen analysis at least 3 months following the procedure and after at least 20 ejaculations.

INTRODUCTION/HISTORY/DEFINITIONS/BACKGROUND

Vasectomy is a safe, effective, and practical option for permanent contraception in men.[1] Vasectomy is a surgical procedure used in men to disrupt and occlude the vas deferens (or vas), which delivers sperm from the testicles. By interrupting sperm transport, this procedure provides permanent sterilization. Vasectomies are typically done under local anesthesia in outpatient settings, and patients usually go home within an hour of the surgery. Surgical techniques used for vasectomy vary widely throughout the world, with limited evidence to guide the most effective approach. Current vasectomy guidelines largely rely on information from observational studies, with few controlled clinical trials.[2]

NATURE OF THE PROBLEM/DIAGNOSIS

Worldwide, more than 40 million men have undergone vasectomy, accounting for about 5% of active contraception.[1] An estimated 527,476 vasectomies were performed in the United States in 2015.[3] Approximately 10% of couples using contraception rely on this method.[1] Roughly 79% of vasectomies in the United States are

Department of Family Medicine, University of North Carolina, 590 Manning Drive, Chapel Hill, NC 27599-7595, USA
* Corresponding author.
E-mail address: mzeitler@med.unc.edu

Prim Care Clin Office Pract 48 (2021) 613–625
https://doi.org/10.1016/j.pop.2021.08.001
0095-4543/21/© 2021 Elsevier Inc. All rights reserved.

performed by urologists, 13% by family physicians, and 8% by general surgeons. From 2007 to 2015, there was a decrease in vasectomies performed in all age groups across the country.[3] Newer data are not available to highlight current trends.

Vasectomies are highly effective, with a failure rate of less than 1% and a low incidence of complications.[1,4] Vasectomy is one of the most cost-effective contraceptive methods available in the United States, next to long-acting reversal contraceptive intrauterine devices. The average cost is $713.00 ($350.00–$1000.00).[5]

A variety of vasectomy techniques are used worldwide, including differing vas isolation methods and vas occlusion techniques (excision and ligation, thermal or electrocautery, and mechanical and chemical occlusion methods), as well as vasectomy with vas irrigation or with fascial interposition.[2]

The best candidates for vasectomy seem to be men older than 30 years in a stable, committed relationship. Younger men, those with partners who work outside the home, and those with a change in marital status following vasectomy are the most likely to eventually request vasectomy reversal.[3,6]

ANATOMY

Knowledge of surgical anatomy is critical to ensure a safe, effective, and efficient vasectomy.

The scrotal skin and spermatic cord are innervated by the ilioinguinal nerve and genital branches of the genitofemoral nerve (**Fig. 1**). Local anesthesia of these nerves provides adequate analgesia for vasectomy.

The layers of tissue beneath the scrotal skin are the dartos fascia and muscle, the external spermatic fascia, and the cremasteric fascia and muscle. The internal spermatic fascia is deep to these structures and covers the spermatic cord, which contains the vas deferens along with its arterial supply (the deferential artery), the pampiniform venous plexus, and the neurovascular supply to testis (**Fig. 2**). The pampiniform plexus

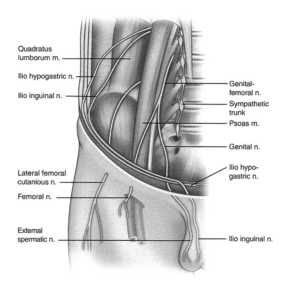

Fig. 1. Scrotal skin and spermatic cord innervation. (*From* Jamnagerwalla J, Kim HH. Groin pain etiology: spermatic cord and testicular causes. In: Jacob BP, Chen DC, Ramshaw B, Towfigh S, eds. The SAGES manual of groin pain. Cham: Springer International Publishing; 2016:111–135.)

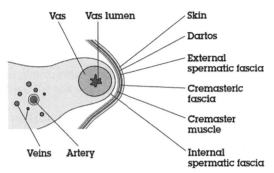

Fig. 2. Surgical anatomy of the scrotum and spermatic cord. (*From* Barone M. Instruments and Supplies. In: No-scalpel Vasectomy: An Illustrated Guide For Surgeons. 3rd ed. Engender-Health; 2002: 15.)

is a network of several veins that lie adjacent to the vas deferens and ultimately drain into the testicular vein. These veins can be easily injured during aggressive dissection of the spermatic cord and cause intraoperative bleeding. Dilatation of the pampiniform plexus, or varicocele, is a common abnormality (more prevalent on the left) that can make isolation of the vas deferens more difficult.

PREOPERATIVE/PREPROCEDURE PLANNING

A preoperative consultation should be conducted, preferably in person. If in-person consultation is not possible, then virtual consultation by telephone, video, or electronic communication is an acceptable alternative.[2]

Before vasectomy, relevant history of abnormalities in sexual development, genital injury, and/or genitourinary surgery should be discussed. In addition, the patient should have a complete genital examination to confirm the presence of a single vas deferens and testicle on each side and absence of anatomic abnormalities that may preclude the procedure or warrant urologic referral. For patients with a history of solitary testicle, extensive genital surgery, or anatomic abnormalities (such as a nonpalpable vas deferens, varicocele, hydrocele, cryptorchidism, or scrotal mass), the surgeon needs to determine whether these complicating factors preclude safe surgery and warrant urologic consultation, or whether the surgeon's surgical skills and experience are adequate to proceed with the vasectomy. Bleeding diathesis may also challenge office-based vasectomy and is another reason to consider referral to a specialist before proceeding.[2]

A preoperative vasectomy consultation should include the following[2]:

- Comprehensive contraception options counseling should be provided.
- Family status should be discussed: relationship status, children (if any), acceptance of procedure by partner, future family intent.
- Ensure understanding of the intended permanence of vasectomy and that the procedure does not produce immediate sterility.
- Following vasectomy, another form of contraception is required until sterility is confirmed by postvasectomy semen analysis (PVSA).
- Even after vas occlusion and sterility are confirmed, vasectomy is not 100% reliable in preventing pregnancy.
- The risk of pregnancy following vasectomy is approximately 1 in 2000 for men who have postvasectomy sterility, defined as azoospermia or PVSA showing rare nonmotile sperm.

- If a technique for vas occlusion known to have a low failure rate is used, then repeat vasectomy is necessary in less than or equal to 1% of patients.
- Patients should refrain from ejaculation for approximately 1 week after vasectomy.
- Options for fertility after vasectomy include vasectomy reversal and sperm retrieval with in vitro fertilization. These options are not always successful and may be expensive.
- The rates of surgical complications such as symptomatic hematoma and postoperative infection are 1% to 2%. These rates vary with the surgeon's experience and the criteria used to diagnose these conditions.
- Chronic scrotal pain, or postvasectomy pain syndrome, occurs after vasectomy in about 1% to 6% of men. Few of these men require additional surgery.
- Other permanent and nonpermanent alternatives to vasectomy are available.
- Recommend ongoing use of condoms to protect against sexually transmitted infections if the patient is not in a committed monogamous relationship.

A thorough preoperative discussion of the procedure by the clinician performing the vasectomy is equally important, and should review the risks, benefits, complications, alternatives, and long-term effects associated with vasectomy. Clinicians do not need to routinely discuss prostate cancer, testicular cancer, coronary heart disease, stroke, hypertension, or dementia in prevasectomy counseling because vasectomy is not a risk factor for these conditions.[2]

Prophylactic antibiotics are not indicated for routine vasectomy unless the patient has a high risk of postoperative infection.[2] Routine preoperative laboratory tests and fasting are also unnecessary.

Contraindications to vasectomy include the presence of a scrotal hematoma, genitourinary or groin infection, and sperm granuloma, but the procedure can often be performed if these issues can be treated and/or resolved.

An anxiolytic, such as diazepam 10 mg orally, can be administered approximately 1 hour before the procedure to help the patient relax and improve surgical isolation of the vas deferens by releasing scrotal and cremasteric muscles. Informed consent must be obtained before anxiolytic administration.

The patient should arrange safe transportation home after the procedure.

PREP AND PATIENT POSITIONING

The temperature of the room is critical because it affects the cremasteric and the scrotal muscles. The room should be warm (21°C–27°C [70°–80° F]), even though a cooler temperature may be more comfortable for the physician.[7]

Application of a topical eutectic mixture of local anesthetic (EMLA) cream reduces the pain of the anesthetic injection when applied 1 hour before incision.[8]

Equipment needed:

- Povidone iodine or chlorhexidine to cleanse the scrotal skin.
- Sterile drapes, sterile gloves, sterile gauze.
- Electrocautery equipment or disposable thermal cautery.
- Sutures (4-0 absorbable, preferably on a noncutting needle).
- A 5-mL to 10-mL syringe with a 38-mm (1.5 inch) 25-gauge or 27-gauge needle for administering local anesthetic.
- Lidocaine 1% or 2% without epinephrine (maximum dose 7 mg/kg [up to 500 mg]).
- Surgical instruments: vas fixation clamp and sharp dissecting forceps, straight scissors, needle holder.

- Surgical clips and surgical clip applier if method of choice for fascial interposition.
- No-needle jet injector if preferred anesthesia technique.
- Other supplies for preferred vasal occlusion method.

The patient is positioned supine on the procedure table. It can be helpful to position and secure the penis onto the lower abdomen with a surgical drape or adhesive tape. Hair is clipped or shaved from the anterior scrotum (either by the surgeon or by the patient before the procedure), which is then prepared with an antiseptic solution. Sterile towels are draped over the area surrounding the scrotum, and sterile technique is used throughout the remainder of the procedure. The vas deferens is then isolated and positioned to lie as superficially as possible beneath the median raphe of the scrotal skin anteriorly, approximately midway between the top of the testes and the base of the penis. This position is usually accomplished using the nondominant hand and a 3-finger technique to manipulate the vas within the scrotum with the middle finger posterior to the vas and the thumb and forefinger anterior. The vas can be digitally grasped between the thumb and middle finger and the forefinger used to stretch the overlying scrotal skin. Local anesthesia can be applied with an external spermatic sheath injection to block the vasal nerve or with a no-needle jet injection technique.[2]

For the vasal nerve block, local anesthetic with or without epinephrine (0.5–1 mL) is injected into the skin to create a wheal over the vas. A large wheal should be avoided because it can distort the scrotal tissue and interfere with isolating the vas. With tension on the vas, the needle is advanced through the anesthetized scrotal skin approximately 2 to 3 cm along the sheath of the vas (but not into the vas) toward the inguinal ring, and 2 to 5 mL of anesthetic is injected into the tissue surrounding the vas; there should not be any resistance. Some operators then anesthetize the contralateral vas to allow ample time for the anesthetic to take effect.[2,9]

The no-needle jet injection technique uses a high-pressure spray to deliver local anesthetic through the scrotal skin and into the tissue surrounding the vas (**Fig. 3**). Caution is indicated because the stream can pass through the patient's tissues and exit with enough force to penetrate the operator's gloved finger. Therefore, the 3-finger technique may need to be modified or the posterior middle fingertip wrapped in tape to ensure operator safety.[2,10,11] A small randomized control trial involving 50 patients showed a statistically significant improvement in pain from anesthetic administration with no-needle vasectomy compared with needle injection. However, there was no statistically significant difference in intraoperative pain between the two techniques.[6,12] The initial cost of the device may be prohibitive.

PROCEDURAL APPROACH

There are 3 key surgical steps in performing vasectomy: (1) isolation of the vas, (2) disruption and occlusion of the vas, and (3) closure of the scrotal skin.

The risks of intraoperative and early postoperative pain, bleeding, and infection are primarily related to the method of vas isolation. The success and failure rates of vasectomy are mainly related to the method of vas occlusion.[2]

Methods of vas isolation include conventional vasectomy and minimally invasive vasectomy, which includes no-scalpel vasectomy.

Conventional vasectomy technique was the most common approach before the introduction of minimally invasive techniques and specialized vasectomy instruments. Conventional vasectomy is performed by making either 1 midline incision or bilateral scrotal incisions using a scalpel. No special instruments are used, and the vas usually is grasped with a towel clip or an Allis forceps. The area of scrotal dissection is

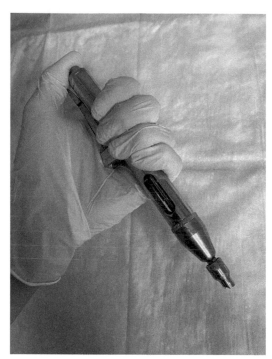

Fig. 3. High-pressure jet injector for delivering local anesthetic spray during the no-needle vasectomy approach.

typically larger than occurs with minimally invasive techniques. This technique accounts for a small proportion of vasectomies performed in the United States but remains the most common technique globally.[2]

The no-scalpel vasectomy technique was developed in 1974 in China by Dr Li Shunqiang and was the first minimally invasive technique for vasectomy. No-scalpel vasectomy is the preferred vasectomy technique in the United States because of its lower complication rates, but it has yet to be adopted worldwide.[2] When combined with the jet injection technique for anesthesia, the surgical approach is termed the no-needle, no-scalpel vasectomy.

Compared with the conventional vasectomy technique, the no-scalpel approach results in less bleeding, hematoma, perioperative pain, and infection, as well as a shorter operation time and a more rapid resumption of sexual activity. Although no difference in vasectomy effectiveness has been shown, sample sizes in studies to date may have been too small to detect differences.[6,13–16]

The no-scalpel vasectomy technique for vas isolation is as follows[2,6,7,13–17]:

1. The vas is positioned under the skin anesthesia wheal using the 3-finger technique described earlier, and a vas fixation ring clamp can be used to gently entrap the vas and a minimal amount of overlying tightly stretched scrotal skin.
2. Apply the vas ring clamp around the vas, perivasal tissue, and overlying skin before making the skin opening (**Fig. 4**).
3. Create a skin opening of less than or equal to 10 mm by piercing the skin with the dissecting forceps or a sharp mosquito hemostat followed by spreading the tissue overlying the vas to expose the bare anterior wall of the vas (see **Fig. 4**). Care

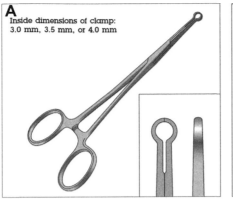
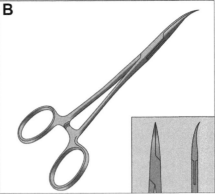

Fig. 4. Ringed clamp (*A*) and dissecting forceps (*B*). (*From* Barone M. Anesthesia. In: No-scalpel Vasectomy: An Illustrated Guide For Surgeons. 3rd ed. EngenderHealth; 2002;7-8.)

should be taken not to go through the vas. An opening approximately twice the width of the vas is made by gently spreading both tips of the hemostat.

4. If a vas fixating clamp is in place, it can be left alone or repositioned as needed.
5. To elevate the vas through the incision, one of 2 methods can be applied:
   a. Pierce or grasp the bare vas with 1 tip of the vas dissector and then use a supination maneuver to elevate the vas above the skin opening.
   b. Grasp the vas through the incision with a different vas ring clamp. The vas can also be elevated through the opening with an Allis clamp or towel clamp.
6. The perivasal tissue is dissected and separated using a dissecting hemostat. Approximately 2 cm of the vas are brought up as a loop. The vas ring clamp can be repositioned at any time for optimal dissection.
7. The loop of vas is cleaned of residual tissue with care to avoid trauma to the perivasal blood vessels. Gauze can be used to achieve finer blunt dissection. Alternatively, the tip of a hemostat or tips of the dissecting forceps can be inserted into the window of the vas deferens loop and gently spread to completely isolate the vas. The vas loop ends can be secured with straight or curved hemostats before excision and end occlusion.
8. The vas is divided and a segment of vas is removed. The minimum length of vas that needs be removed to prevent recanalization and possible vasectomy failure is controversial. Recanalization rates more likely reflect occlusion technique than the length of vas segment removed.[18] Typically, removal of at least 10 to 15 mm is favored, but this varies in practice between 0 and 5 cm.[2,18]
9. If a segment is removed, it can be sent for pathologic confirmation. However, routine histologic examination of the excised vas segments is not required. Histologic documentation that full-thickness vas was excised can be helpful in the event of vasectomy failure.
10. Occlude the vas with the surgeon's preferred technique for vas occlusion, discussed later.
11. Scrotal closure by preferred technique as described later.

Vasal Occlusion Methods

Vasal disruption and subsequent occlusion can be accomplished in multiple ways, and methods for managing the testicular vasal end are debated. Simple suture ligation with excision is the most common method worldwide, although it has been shown to be less effective because of likely vasal end ischemic necrosis and sloughing, which can lead to spontaneous recanalization.[14,19] In this method, the vas is occluded with ligatures or clips and the vas excised between the occluded points. The number of ligatures on each end of the divided vas varies, as does the length of the segment excised. Folding back is a technique of folding and suturing each divided vas end on itself to prevent the 2 cut ends from facing each other. Ligation and excision should not be used as the sole method of vasal disruption given failure rates as high as 1% to 6%.[2,14]

Mucosal cautery is the technique of applying thermal or electrical cautery to the mucosa of the cut ends of the vas to destroy the vasal mucosa, creating scar tissue to occlude the vas lumen. The length of the cauterized segment varies from a few millimeters to 1.5 cm. Cautery may be combined with excision of a vas segment, folding back, or fascial interposition.[2] Thermal cautery or electrocautery of the vas lumen is more effective than ligation and excision alone.[15] Fulguration using a battery-powered handheld cautery (red-hot wire) seems to scar and occlude the vas lumen more effectively than electrocautery.[19,20] Inexpensive, battery-powered thermal cautery devices are commercially available.[15]

Intraluminal cautery without separation of the vasa is the preferred method practiced at Marie Stopes International health centers (multinational family planning clinics where 100,000 vasectomies have been performed worldwide), with a reported failure rate less than 1%.[2,21,22] The technique was developed to be easily disseminated across global health settings but is not commonly performed in the United States.

Irrigation of the vas with saline or spermicidal agents does not have any documented benefit. Three randomized trials failed to show any acceleration of sperm clearance and sterility by irrigation of the prostatic end during vasectomy.[4,23–25]

Fascial interposition is the technique of burying 1 vasal end within the internal spermatic fascia to separate the anatomic plane between the 2 vasal ends, minimizing the risk of recanalization.[6] The fascial layer may be placed over the testicular or the abdominal end.

A clip or absorbable suture is used to tack a layer of the vas sheath between the 2 cut vasal ends. Fascial interposition significantly reduces vasectomy failure compared with no fascial interposition (odds ratio, 0.42; 95% confidence interval, 0.26–0.70). However, it lengthens the procedure by 2 to 3 minutes. For men younger than 30 years, fascial interposition also increased the likelihood of azoospermia.[4,26] The fascial layer may be placed over the testicular or the abdominal/prostatic end. Typically, fascial interposition is combined with other techniques such as ligation and excision or mucosal cautery.

Recent evidence suggests that cautery plus fascial interposition is more effective than ligation and excision plus fascial interposition, with a failure rate as low as 0.3% in 1 study.[15,27] Another study showed the efficacy of the combined approach (thermal cautery of both ends and fascial interposition) with no failures (ie, pregnancies) and a low rate of complications (congestive epididymitis in 4.8%, sperm granuloma in 1.4%).[28] In the Unites States, this is the preferred method for vasal occlusion.

Open-ended vasectomy is the technique of leaving the testicular end of the divided vas unoccluded while occluding the abdominal/prostatic end. This technique offers the theoretic advantage of decreasing postvasectomy vasal pressure, congestive epididymitis, and painful sperm granuloma formation. When open-ended vasectomy is performed, fascial interposition is typically used to prevent recanalization.[29] The open-ended technique can be offered to the patient. However, most men choose to have both vasal ends occluded.

In addition, care should be taken intraoperatively to ensure that 1 vas is not occluded twice. For a single-incision or no-scalpel vasectomy, the surgeon should ensure that the same vas is not isolated and occluded in 2 locations, leaving the other vas unoccluded. A gentle tug on each vas during isolation causes the ipsilateral testis to move, which can help ensure bilateral vasal disruption and occlusion.

Scrotal closure can be accomplished with clips, clamps, sutures, or cyanoacrylate tissue adhesive (surgical glue or Dermabond). The incision also may be left open to heal by secondary intention. Data comparing these methods are limited.[14] Once the procedure is completed, the wound can be covered with a sterile dressing. The patient is assisted in putting on tight-fitting underwear or scrotal support.

COMPLICATIONS

Bleeding and hematoma formation are the most common complications of vasectomy, often resulting from injury to the pampiniform venous plexus. Perioperative bleeding occurs in 2.4% of no-scalpel vasectomies and 4.0% of conventional vasectomies, whereas hematoma occurs in 2.4% of no-scalpel vasectomies and 12.5% of conventional vasectomies. In rare cases, bleeding may be severe enough to require surgical intervention, such as scrotal exploration, hematoma evacuation, and control of bleeding. Postoperative infection occurs in 0.7% of no-scalpel vasectomies and 2.2% of conventional vasectomies.[6,13,30]

A sperm granuloma may form as an immunologic reaction to the extravasation of highly antigenic sperm from the testicular vasal end. Sperm may leak from the testicular side of an open-ended vas or from a cauterized or fulgurated vas. Although most sperm granulomas are not painful and often involute over time, they may play a role in postvasectomy pain syndrome and recanalization with vasectomy failure.[6,13,14,30]

Postvasectomy pain syndrome, distinct from postprocedure pain, is persistent or recurrent scrotal pain that occurs months to years after vasectomy. It is thought to be caused by chronic epididymal congestion, with an incidence between 1% and 6%. Mild postvasectomy pain syndrome is treated symptomatically with acetaminophen, nonsteroidal antiinflammatory medications, and warm baths. If unsuccessful, local nerve blocks or steroid injections may be performed by a pain specialist. If the pain is localized to a palpable granuloma, this may be excised, followed by fulguration of the leaking end of the vas. Severe or intractable cases may require surgical intervention, including either vasectomy reversal or complete epididymectomy.[6,13,14,30]

RECOVERY AND REHABILITATION (INCLUDING POSTPROCEDURE CARE)

The dressing and scrotal support are maintained for 48 to 72 hours after surgery. Applying an ice pack intermittently to the scrotum for 24 to 48 hours can help decrease discomfort and swelling. Postprocedure pain varies with the vasectomy technique and surgeon experience and is usually self-limited. Acetaminophen or nonsteroidal antiinflammatory medications along with ice usually provide sufficient analgesia, although occasionally narcotic analgesics may be necessary.

Postoperative instructions should be reviewed with the patient. Mild pain, swelling, and bruising are expected for the first 2 to 3 days. The patient should call for increasing pain, bleeding from the incision site, fever, scrotal redness, discharge, or significant swelling.

Bed rest is typically recommended for the first 24 hours following a vasectomy. The patient may return to gentle activity on postoperative day 1 and light work in 2 to 3 days but should refrain from heavy work, sports, or lifting for 1 week. Sexual activity and ejaculation are avoided for 1 week. Vasectomy does not produce immediate sterility. After vasectomy, sperm can survive in the vas or seminal vesicles for several months, so another form of contraceptive must be used until sterility is verified by postvasectomy semen analysis (PVSA), typically obtained at 12 weeks postprocedure.

MANAGEMENT

Azoospermia is the ideal end point of vasectomy and definitive evidence of sterility. One PVSA showing azoospermia performed after 3 months and 20 ejaculations is sufficient to establish sterility. According to the World Health Organization, the semen sample should be obtained after a period of abstinence of 2 to 7 days, kept at body temperature, transported within 60 minutes of collection, and analyzed in the laboratory within 4 hours of ejaculation. A metanalysis of 56 studies suggested that approximately 80% of patients achieve azoospermia 3 months after vasectomy and after 11 to 20 ejaculations. A small percentage of patients (1.4%) showed persistent presence of nonmotile sperm, although some of them eventually achieved azoospermia.[31] Time to azoospermia decreases with increasing number of ejaculations and coital frequency following vasectomy and increases with patient age.[32]

The British Andrology Society recommends that patients with presence of persistent nonmotile sperm on PVSA undergo monthly follow-up samples until 1 test shows azoospermia or 2 consecutive tests show low numbers of nonmotile sperm (<100,000/mL) and 7 months have elapsed since vasectomy. The latter group may also stop using alternative contraception because the continued presence of rare, nonmotile sperm is probably clinically insignificant and probability of pregnancy is extremely low.[33] The American Urologic Association guidelines state that patients may stop using other methods of contraception when examination of 1 well-mixed, uncentrifuged, fresh postvasectomy semen specimen shows azoospermia or only rare nonmotile sperm (defined as presence of ≤100,000 nonmotile sperm per milliliter based on microscopic examination of at least 50 high-power fields [HPFs]).[2]

In the United States, the Clinical Laboratory Improvement Act (CLIA) distinguishes provider-performed microscopy analysis from that in laboratories performing more complex testing. These regulations allow for semen analysis in a doctor's office if the reported result is qualitative (ie, limited to the presence or absence of sperm and detection of motility). Thus, physicians are permitted to conduct PVSA in their offices, but they are not allowed to determine sperm concentration unless the office laboratory has a high-complexity level of CLIA certification. There is interest in developing a method of estimating the number of sperm per milliliter of semen from the number of sperm per HPF found in a PVSA. Such a method would allow physicians to correlate the number of sperm per HPF in PVSAs that do not show azoospermia to various concentrations of sperm per milliliter and more readily make guideline-based recommendations.

Compliance with PVSA is a common issue, with a median of 19% of patients failing to provide any sample and 5% only partially complying with collection instructions.[6] In response to noncompliance, a novel, qualitative home test has been developed that can accurately detect sperm counts less than 250,000/mL (positive predictive value, 93%; negative predictive value, 97%). Although approved by the US Food and Drug Administration, this test cannot assess sperm motility and is not yet supported by clinical trials or current guidelines to confirm sterility.[2,6]

OUTCOMES

The proportion of vasectomies that fail (defined as lack of azoospermia on semen analysis or presence of pregnancy) is generally considered to be between zero and

2%, with most studies reporting a failure rate of less than 1%.[4] Vasectomy failure can be caused by technical errors, recanalization, unprotected intercourse before azoospermia is documented, or, in rare cases, aberrant anatomy such as a redundant/ accessory vas. Recanalization following vasectomy is rare (0.4%) and pregnancy is even rarer (0.07%).[34] The presence of motile spermatozoa during the 3-month postvasectomy semen analysis likely represents vasectomy failure and should be confirmed with another semen analysis 1 month later. Once motile spermatozoa are reconfirmed, repeat vasectomy is recommended if desired by the patient.

Some men may be concerned that vasectomy is linked to prostate cancer or testicular cancer. Studies have shown that there is no measurable association between vasectomy and malignancy of the prostate or testes.[6,14]

Although vasectomy should be performed only for patients desiring permanent sterility, decisions regarding fertility and family planning may change. Vasectomy can be reversed with microsurgical techniques, which have varying success rates. Vasectomy reversal involves reanastomosis (vasovasostomy) of the vas deferens, ideally at the site of the previous disruption and occlusion. Successful vasectomy reversal has been reported in 50% to 70% of men. Rates decline with increasing time between vasectomy and reversal.[35–37] Two important positive predictors of success are time since vasectomy (<15 years) and age of female partner (<40 years).[6]

CLINICS CARE POINTS

- Vasectomy is an accessible, safe, efficacious, and cost-effective option for permanent contraception in men.
- Diazepam 10 mg orally 1 hour before the procedure as well as topical EMLA cream applied to the anterior scrotum may reduce anxiety and pain related to the procedure.
- The no-needle jet injection technique is preferred for anesthesia if available. If not, local vasal nerve blockade should be used.
- The preferred method for vas deferens isolation with lowest complication rate is the minimally invasive, no-scalpel technique with a ring clamp and dissecting forceps.
- The preferred occlusion method with optimal success rate is vasal excision with end cauterization and fascial interposition of the prostatic/abdominal end. This method has the lowest failure rate.
- One postvasectomy semen analysis showing azoospermia performed after 3 months and 20 ejaculations is sufficient to establish sterility.
- Some men may have persistent nonmotile sperm, which is likely clinically insignificant if confirmed on multiple sperm analysis and if there are less than 100,000 sperm/mL. These patients may cautiously stop alternative forms of contraception.
- Vasectomy reversal is possible, with varying success rates.

REFERENCES

1. Page ST, Amory JK, Bremner WJ. Advances in male contraception. Endocr Rev 2008;29(4):465–93.
2. Sharlip ID, Belker AM, Honig S, et al. Vasectomy: AUA guideline. J Urol 2012; 188(6 Suppl):2482–91.
3. Ostrowski KA, Holt SK, Haynes B, et al. Evaluation of vasectomy trends in the united states. Urology 2018;118:76–9.

4. Cook LA, Van Vliet HAAM, Lopez LM, et al. Vasectomy occlusion techniques for male sterilization. Cochrane Database Syst Rev 2014;(3):CD003991.

5. Trussell J, Lalla AM, Doan QV, et al. Cost effectiveness of contraceptives in the United States. Contraception 2009;79(1):5–14.

6. Rayala BZ, Viera AJ. Common questions about vasectomy. Am Fam Physician 2013;88(11):757–61.

7. Barone M. No-scalpel vasectomy: an illustrated guide for surgeons. 3rd edition. A V S C Intl; 2003 EngenderHealth. ISBN: 1-885063-34-2.

8. Cooper TP. Use of EMLA cream with vasectomy. Urology 2002;60(1):135–7.

9. Li PS, Li SQ, Schlegel PN, et al. External spermatic sheath injection for vasal nerve block. Urology 1992;39(2):173–6.

10. Weiss RS, Li PS. No-needle jet anesthetic technique for no-scalpel vasectomy. J Urol 2005;173(5):1677–80.

11. Wilson CL. No-needle anesthetic for no-scalpel vasectomy. Am Fam Physician 2001;63(7):1295.

12. White MA, Maatman TJ. Comparative analysis of effectiveness of two local anesthetic techniques in men undergoing no-scalpel vasectomy. Urology 2007;70(6): 1187–9.

13. Cook LA, Pun A, Gallo MF, et al. Scalpel versus no-scalpel incision for vasectomy. Cochrane Database Syst Rev 2014;(3):CD004112.

14. Dassow P, Bennett JM. Vasectomy: an update. Am Fam Physician 2006;74(12): 2069–74.

15. Aradhya KW, Best K, Sokal DC. Recent developments in vasectomy. BMJ 2005; 330(7486):296–9.

16. Clenney TL, Higgins JC. Vasectomy techniques. Am Fam Physician 1999; 60(1):151.

17. Sokal D, McMullen S, Gates D, et al. A comparative study of the no scalpel and standard incision approaches to vasectomy in 5 countries. The Male Sterilization Investigator Team. J Urol 1999;162(5):1621–5.

18. Labrecque M, Hoang D-Q, Turcot L. Association between the length of the vas deferens excised during vasectomy and the risk of postvasectomy recanalization. Fertil Steril 2003;79(4):1003–7.

19. Denniston GC. Vasectomy by electrocautery: outcomes in a series of 2,500 patients. J Fam Pract 1985;21(1):35–40.

20. Schmidt SS, Minckler TM. The vas after vasectomy: comparison of cauterization methods. Urology 1992;40(5):468–70.

21. Black T, Francome C. The evolution of the Marie Stopes electrocautery no-scalpel vasectomy procedure. J Fam Plann Reprod Health Care 2002;28(3):137–8.

22. Black TR, Gates DS, Lavely K, et al. The percutaneous electrocoagulation vasectomy technique–a comparative trial with the standard incision technique at Marie Stopes House, London. Contraception 1989;39(4):359–68.

23. Pearce I, Adeyoju A, Bhatt RI, et al. The effect of perioperative distal vasal lavage on subsequent semen analysis after vasectomy: a prospective randomized controlled trial. BJU Int 2002;90(3):282–5.

24. Eisner B, Schuster T, Rodgers P, et al. A randomized clinical trial of the effect of intraoperative saline perfusion on postvasectomy azoospermia. Ann Fam Med 2004;2(3):221–3.

25. Mason RG, Dodds L, Swami SK. Sterile water irrigation of the distal vas deferens at vasectomy: does it accelerate clearance of sperm? A prospective randomized trial. Urology 2002;59(3):424–7.

26. Cook LA, Van Vliet H, Lopez LM, et al. Vasectomy occlusion techniques for male sterilization. Cochrane Database Syst Rev 2007;(2):CD003991.
27. Sokal D, Irsula B, Chen-Mok M, et al. A comparison of vas occlusion techniques: cautery more effective than ligation and excision with fascial interposition. BMC Urol 2004;4(1):12.
28. Schmidt SS. Vasectomy by section, luminal fulguration and fascial interposition: results from 6248 cases. Br J Urol 1995;76(3):373–4 [discussion: 375].
29. Labrecque M, Nazerali H, Mondor M, et al. Effectiveness and complications associated with 2 vasectomy occlusion techniques. J Urol 2002;168(6):2495–8 [discussion: 2498].
30. Cook LA, Pun A, van Vliet H, et al. Scalpel versus no-scalpel incision for vasectomy. Cochrane Database Syst Rev 2007;(2):CD004112.
31. Griffin T, Tooher R, Nowakowski K, et al. How little is enough? The evidence for post-vasectomy testing. J Urol 2005;174(1):29–36.
32. Arango Toro O, Andolz Peitivi P, Lladó Carbonell C, et al. [Post-vasectomy semen in 313 males. Statistical analysis, medical aspects, legal implications]. Arch Esp Urol 1993;46(1):29–34.
33. Hancock P, McLaughlin E, British Andrology Society. British Andrology Society guidelines for the assessment of post vasectomy semen samples (2002). J Clin Pathol 2002;55(11):812–6.
34. Jamieson DJ, Costello C, Trussell J, et al. The risk of pregnancy after vasectomy. Obstet Gynecol 2004;103(5 Pt 1):848–50.
35. Belker AM, Thomas AJ, Fuchs EF, et al. Results of 1,469 microsurgical vasectomy reversals by the Vasovasostomy Study Group. J Urol 1991;145(3):505–11.
36. Sharlip ID. What is the best pregnancy rate that may be expected from vasectomy reversal? J Urol 1993;149(6):1469–71.
37. Hendry WF. Vasectomy and vasectomy reversal. Br J Urol 1994;73(4):337–44.

Performance and Interpretation of Office Exercise Stress Testing

Heath C. Thornton, MD, CAQSM*, Fadi Hanna, MD, Kiran Mullur, MD

KEYWORDS

- Stress testing • Cardiac test • Treadmill • Exercise • Coronary disease
- Electrocardiography

KEY POINTS

- Exercise electrocardiogram (ECG) stress testing is a cost-effective, accurate, and patient-centered diagnostic tool for patients suspected of having stable ischemic heart disease.
- Calculating pretest probability is a critical step in determining appropriateness of exercise ECG stress testing.
- Appropriate equipment, staffing, and training is required to properly and safely conduct and interpret clinic-based exercise stress testing.
- Exercise ECG stress testing incorporates objective and subjective parameters that are strong predictors of cardiovascular disease, including ST-segment changes, ischemic symptoms, exercise tolerance, arrhythmia induction, and hemodynamic responses.

INTRODUCTION

Coronary artery disease (CAD) continues to be a leading cause of death and disability in adults in developed countries. CAD resulted in over 7 million deaths globally in 2010 and accounts for nearly 600,000 deaths in the United States every year.[1,2] Despite mortality from CAD gradually declining in Western countries, the 2016 Heart Disease and Stroke Statistics update of the American Heart Association (AHA) reported that 15.5 million people in the US older than 20 years have CAD.[3–5] The costs of caring for patients with CAD are enormous; estimated at $156 billion in the United States for 2008.[1] While 1% of all ambulatory primary care office visits are for chest pain, only 2% to 4% of those patients will have unstable angina or an acute myocardial infarction.[6] The clinician is challenged with distinguishing the more serious etiologies of chest pain while not overtesting and overtreating the nonworrisome causes. Outpatient exercise ECG stress testing is a useful clinical tool to meet that challenge.

Department of Family and Community Medicine, Wake Forest School of Medicine, Medical Center Boulevard, Winston-Salem, NC 27157-1084, USA
* Corresponding author.
E-mail address: hthornto@wakehealth.edu

Prim Care Clin Office Pract 48 (2021) 627–643
https://doi.org/10.1016/j.pop.2021.07.009
0095-4543/21/© 2021 Elsevier Inc. All rights reserved.

primarycare.theclinics.com

With CAD and myocardial ischemia, there is a physiologic mismatch between myocardial oxygen demand and the ability of a stenosed artery to supply oxygenated blood to the exercising myocardium. The essence of the exercise stress test is to intensify this mismatch, thereby leading to myocardial ischemia symptoms, ECG changes, and hemodynamic changes in heart rate (HR) and blood pressure (BP). These factors, combined with assessment of exercise functional capacity, are strong predictors for the presence of CAD and all-cause mortality.[1]

Stress Testing Modalities

While stress testing can be performed in a variety of ways, the most used and widely available stress testing modalities are exercise electrocardiography, exercise echocardiography, and pharmacologic stress cardiac imaging (echocardiography or radionuclide myocardial perfusion imaging [MPI]). As a result of significant advances in computed tomography, cardiac magnetic resonance imaging, and echocardiography, assessments of CAD and myocardial ischemia are both highly sensitive and specific.[7] However, these advances have also resulted in an increase in the number of noninvasive radionuclide and echocardiographic imaging studies performed to identify CAD. More than 9 million MPI studies were performed in 2008 at a cost of >$1 billion and significant radiation exposure.[8] As the US faces both increasing health care costs and increasing prevalence of cardiovascular disease, there is a need for careful allocation of limited resources.[8] Furthermore, when caring for patients with suspected CAD, physicians must consider testing that is patient-centered. This involves considering a test's risk profile and cost-effectiveness and not simply its diagnostic accuracy.

Exercise electrocardiography has a long history of use for CAD diagnosis and prognostication.[3] When performed in the outpatient setting, exercise stress testing decreases the cost associated with hospitalization without worsening patient outcomes.[9] A 2006 randomized trial of 457 patients found that exercise ECG testing was more cost-effective than MPI in patients with lower probability of CAD.[10] Using physical activity, the physiologic conditions which trigger the patient's presenting symptoms are mimicked. Exercise ECG changes combined with other clinical parameters obtained during the test can both reliably predict CAD, helping to guide further management, and reliably rule out CAD, preventing unnecessary interventions.[8] The sensitivity and specificity of exercise stress testing for the detection of CAD are approximately 68% and 77%, respectively.[11] The study also offers a reassuring safety profile, with a peri-procedural death rate of approximately 0.01%.[12] Symptom-limited exercise testing is the preferred form of stress for patients who can attain an adequate level of exercise because it provides the most information about patients' symptoms and their hemodynamic response during exercise.[9]

Pretest Probability

Once a physician determines that a patient's presentation may represent obstructive CAD, the patient's overall risk of CAD can be designated as either low, moderate, or high. This stratification allows for selection of the best diagnostic study to evaluate the patient's presenting symptoms. There are several risk algorithms available that can be used to calculate pretest probability of obstructive CAD. Both the American College of Cardiology (ACC) and the European Society of Cardiology recommend that clinicians stratify patient risk for CAD based on age, sex, and quality of chest pain.[13–15] The ACC guidelines are shown in **Table 1**. Typical chest pain is defined as (1) deep, poorly localized chest or arm discomfort (pain or pressure), (2) associated with physical exertion or

Table 1
Pretest probability of coronary artery disease by age, gender, and symptoms[a]

Age (y)	Gender	Typical/ Definite Angina Pectoris	Atypical/ Probable Angina Pectoris	Nonanginal Chest Pain	Asymptomatic
30–39	Men	Intermediate	Intermediate	Low	Very low
	Women	Intermediate	Very low	Very low	Very low
40–49	Men	High	Intermediate	Intermediate	Low
	Women	Intermediate	Low	Very low	Very low
50–59	Men	High	Intermediate	Intermediate	Low
	Women	Intermediate	Intermediate	Low	Very low
60–69	Men	High	Intermediate	Intermediate	Low
	Women	High	Intermediate	Intermediate	Low

[a] No data exist for patients younger than 30 y or older than 69 y, but it can be assumed that prevalence of CAD increases with age. In a few cases, patients with ages at the extremes of the decades listed may have probabilities slightly outside the high or low range. High indicates greater than 90%; intermediate, 10%–90%; low, less than 10%; and very low, less than 5%.

From Gibbons RJ, Balady GJ, Bricker JT, Chaitman BR, Fletcher GF, Froelicher VF, Mark DB, McCallister BD, Mooss AN, O'Reilly MG, Winters WL Jr. ACC/AHA 2002 guideline update for exercise testing: summary article: a report of the ACC/AHA Task Force on Practice Guidelines (Committee to Update the 1997 Exercise Testing Guidelines). J Am Coll Cardiol 2002;40:1531–40.

emotional stress, and (3) relieved with rest or sublingual nitroglycerin within 5 minutes.[9] Atypical chest pain has two of the three characteristics, while nonanginal chest pain may have one or none.[9]

Indications and Contraindications

According to the ACC/AHA, for patients who present with an intermediate pretest probability of CAD, exercise stress testing should be considered as a first-line diagnostic test, assuming adequate exercise tolerance and normal resting ECG.[7] Select indications for exercise ECG stress testing pertinent for the outpatient clinic setting are listed in **Box 1**.

It is also important to understand the limitations of exercise stress testing. Some conditions, ECG findings, and functional limitations can increase the likelihood of a nondiagnostic exercise ECG test or create undue risk to the patient (**Box 2**).

Preprocedural Planning

Each potential candidate for testing should be evaluated by a medical provider for proper indications (see **Box 1**) and relevant contraindications (see **Box 2**). A thorough history and clinical examination should be performed and documented by the referring provider or testing provider. A resting ECG should be performed. Documentation should explicitly identify

- Indication(s) for testing
- Absence of contraindications. Presence of relative contraindications and reasons why proceeding with testing is still warranted
- Interpretation of resting ECG
- Medications (especially those that might affect physiologic response to exercise)
- Ability to perform the exercise component of the testing

Box 1
Indications for exercise EKG stress testing

Diagnosis
- Patients with chest pain syndrome or symptom equivalent[9]
  - Intermediate risk (class I recommendation)[2]
  - Low risk (class IIa recommendation)[2]
- Patients with known stable CAD with stable angina, new or worsening symptoms[2]
- Exercise-associated syncope/presyncope after other appropriate workup
- Interval screening of known stable ischemic heart disease in patients with prior "silent ischemia" or high risk for cardiac event[2]

Prognosis (risk assessment)
- Patient with known stable Ischemic Heart Disease (IHD)[2,13]
- Patients with suspected stable IHD[13]
- Asymptomatic patient with Diabetes Mellitus starting vigorous exercise program[13]
- Asymptomatic patient with multiple risk factors for risk reduction plan[13]
- Asymptomatic men (>45 y) and women (>55 y)[13]
  - Starting vigorous exercise
  - High risk of CAD due to other medical conditions
  - High risk occupations to public safety

Physiologic response to exercise
- Exercise capacity[9]
- Hypertension[13]
- Chronotropic competence[9]

Box 2
Contraindications to exercise testing

Absolute
- Acute myocardial infarction (within 2 d)
- Unstable angina not previously stabilized by medical therapy
- Uncontrolled cardiac arrhythmias causing symptoms or hemodynamic compromise
- Symptomatic severe aortic stenosis
- Uncontrolled symptomatic heart failure
- Acute pulmonary embolus or pulmonary infarction
- Acute myocarditis or pericarditis
- Acute aortic dissection

Relative[a]
- Left main coronary stenosis
- Moderate stenotic valvular heart disease
- Electrolyte abnormalities
- Severe arterial hypertension[b]
- Tachyarrhythmias or bradyarrhythmias
- Hypertrophic cardiomyopathy and other forms of outflow tract obstruction
- Mental or physical impairment leading to inability to exercise adequately
- High-degree atrioventricular block

[a]Relative contraindications can be superseded if the benefits of exercise outweigh the risks.[b]In the absence of definitive evidence, the committee suggests systolic blood pressure of greater than 200 mm Hg and/or diastolic blood pressure of greater than 110 mm Hg.

From Gibbons RJ, Balady GJ, Bricker JT, Chaitman BR, Fletcher GF, Froelicher VF, Mark DB, McCallister BD, Mooss AN, O'Reilly MG, Winters WL Jr. ACC/AHA 2002 guideline update for exercise testing: summary article: a report of the ACC/AHA Task Force on Practice Guidelines (Committee to Update the 1997 Exercise Testing Guidelines). J Am Coll Cardiol 2002;40:1531–40.

Selection of Testing Method

There are several modes of performing exercise ECG stress testing. While the most common is motorized treadmill, the stationary cycle ergometer and arm ergometer are also been used. The pros and cons of each are listed in **Table 2**. A patient's capacity to exercise is often predicted in an informal manner based on his or her reported activity level. If a person can walk for more than 5 minutes on flat ground or up one to two flights of stairs without needing to stop, that person most likely can achieve an adequate workload during exercise stress testing.[17] For those individuals able to ambulate safely for 10 minutes, a treadmill-based exercise test is generally preferred.

Beta-Blockers and Exercise

There has been much discussion regarding the advantages and disadvantages of holding beta-adrenergic receptor antagonist medications for stress testing. This class of medications attenuates the HR and BP response to exercise and has potential effects on exercise capacity. Data and research reports, however, have been inconclusive regarding beta-blocker medications' effect on testing outcomes and diagnostic accuracy.[13,18] The clinician performing the exercise stress test should evaluate the risk of stopping a beta-blocker before the procedure compared with the potential reduction in sensitivity and specificity of the test.[9,13] This decision should be documented in the stress test report. If the medication is continued, interpretation of the testing results should account for its effect.

Instructions to Patient

The purpose and process of the test should be thoroughly explained to the patient before the procedure. Recommended instructions include

- Wear appropriate clothing and shoes for exercise,
- Maintain adequate oral hydration,
- Hold medications, if any,
- Avoid food for 3 hours before testing,
- Avoid caffeine for 24 hours before testing,
- Avoid tobacco use for 24 hours before testing.

Equipment and Staffing

Essential equipment for testing in an outpatient office setting includes

- ECG machine with continuous monitoring and on-demand printing capability

Table 2
Pros and cons of exercise testing modalities

Modality	Pros	Cons
Treadmill	Consistent speed Simulates common activity Variety of protocols to customize to patient Higher peak Vo_2	Treadmill dictates speed Risk of falls Gait/balance problems Weight capacity limit
Cycle ergometer	Low risk of falls More comfortable for those with gait/balance problems Higher weight capacity	Must maintain pedal speed Foot positioning on pedals Lower peak Vo_2[16]
Arm ergometer	For those with lower limb disabilities[16]	Uncommon arm movement Lower work rates, peak Vo_2[16]

- Electrodes compatible with ECG cables
- BP monitor, ideally automated
- Treadmill with incline grade adjustment capability (or cycle ergometer/arm ergometer)
- Pulse oximeter
- Automatic external defibrillator or manual external defibrillator
- Cardiac resuscitation medications and supplies
- Oxygen

There are numerous stress test systems on the market with integrated ECG monitoring and treadmill devices. These systems allow for automated incline and speed changes based on chosen protocol, automated ECG printing at predetermined intervals, documentation of patient measurements, integration with electronic medical records, and a printed report of the completed test. Some systems integrate automated BP and pulse oximetry measurements. Front and side rails are highly recommended to increase patient safety. These features enhance the provider's ability to focus on monitoring ECG and patient status changes during testing and recovery.

Appropriately trained personnel are critical for proper administration of the outpatient exercise stress test. Medical providers and staff should all be trained in Basic Life Support and Advanced Cardiac Life Support protocols. Familiarity with onsite resuscitation equipment and supplies and their locations should be established before testing. The medical provider should be familiar with testing equipment and have training and knowledge consistent with recommended guidelines for stress testing.[19,20] Staff should have skills and knowledge specific to their assigned roles. This includes ECG electrode placement, equipment management and use, and obtaining BP measurement while the patient is exercising. Clear, concise communication between testing team members augments the efficiency and safety of the procedure.

Prep and Patient Positioning

On the day of the procedure, staff should obtain vital signs including supine BP and pulse. The medical provider should perform a brief review of history and physical examination. This will allow for identification of missed or new contraindications. Consent for the procedure should be obtained by reviewing the purpose and process of the study. Discussion of the risks and benefits associated with exercise stress testing should include those noted in **Box 3**. Consent forms should be signed by the patient and witness.

Then, the target heart rate (THR) is calculated to determine the HR threshold for an adequate test. Multiple calculations have been studied and validated in the literature. All are designed to accurately approximate the patient's physiologic maximal HR. The THR is typically considered 85% of the maximum predicted heart rate (MPHR) and may be calculated as THR = (220 – age) × 0.85. While HR has a predictable linear rise with exercise and is highly influenced by age changes, there is still significant variability in maximum HR within the same age group. Therefore, THR should not be used as the sole determinant of adequate effort.[9] Termination of the stress test based on THR alone may limit the evaluation of exercise capacity and mortality prognosis. Sensitivity of the exercise stress test increases when the patient exceeds the calculated THR.[9,21]

Finally, the patient's skin is prepared for electrode placement. To reduce impedance and artifact, shave body hair and clean the skin with alcohol at electrode placement sites. Precordial lead placement is identical to that for resting ECG. Limb lead placement, however, is altered because of anticipated extremity movement during testing (**Fig. 1**).

Box 3
Risks and complications associated with exercise stress testing

Cardiovascular
- Arrhythmias
- Acute coronary syndrome
- Hypotension
- Hypertensive response
- Syncope
- Death (rare)

Musculoskeletal
- Sprains/strains
- Muscle cramps/soreness
- Joint pain
- Fractures
- Contusions

General
- Fatigue
- Lightheadedness
- Dehydration
- Shortness of breath

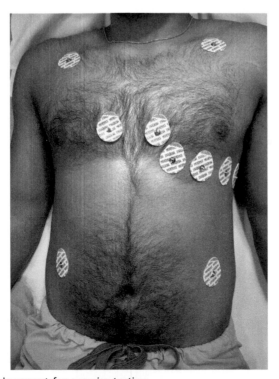

Fig. 1. ECG lead placement for exercise testing.

Procedural Approach

The exercise stress protocol is selected based on the goals of testing and on the estimated functional capacity of the patient. There are numerous protocols designed to systematically increase patient workload by increasing treadmill incline and/or speed. The Bruce protocol is widely known and often used because of its familiarity with clinicians and evidence base. Because it has large changes in workload between stages, the Bruce protocol may not be tolerated by patients with functional limitations and limited exercise capacity. Testing protocols that use constant treadmill speed or consistent treadmill incline may be better suited for patients with different limitations. Comparison of multiple protocols is available in other publications.[21]

During each stage, the patient's BP, HR, ECG, symptoms, and perceived workload should be documented. Rating of perceived exertion (RPE), measured with the Borg scale (**Box 4**), allows for patient-directed measurement of overall physical exertion and fatigue. While this patient metric is subjective and is influenced by multiple factors, it does have utility in judging exercise effort and testing adequacy when combined with THR.[9,22,23]

The following is an example of procedural steps.

Pretest Stages

- Obtain supine resting EKG: last review for contraindications to testing
- Transfer patient to stationary treadmill and obtain standing baseline EKG, BP, and pulse.
- Discuss safety on treadmill (stay toward the front of the machine, wait for treadmill to be stopped, and so forth) and emergency stop button
- Review testing protocol (speed, incline changes per protocol) and measurements (BP, RPE score)
- Review goal for adequate test (ie, THR and RPE goals) and patient's ability to determine when the test is terminated
- Allow time for patient to ask questions before initiating test

---

Box 4
The 15-grade scale for ratings of perceived exertion, the RPE scale

6	
7	Very, very light
8	
9	Very light
10	
11	Fairly light
12	
13	Somewhat hard
14	
15	Hard
16	
17	Very hard
18	
19	Very, very hard
20	

From Borg, GA. Psychophysical bases of perceived exertion. Med Sci Sports Exerc 1982; 14(5): 377-381.

Exercise Stages

- During each stage:
  - Obtain and record BP
  - Print EKG toward the end of stage (frequently automated)
  - Record RPE score
  - Record absence or presence of clinical symptoms
  - Notify patient of change in upcoming stage elevation and/or speed
- Monitor for indications for termination of the study (**Box 5**)
- Once the decision for termination of exercise has been made:
  - Verbalize to patient the intention to discontinue exercise
  - Notify briefly of recovery phase expectations

Recovery Stages

- Immediately after exercise
  - Print ECG
  - Ask the patient to identify most significant reason for terminating test if the test was terminated because of patient request
  - Obtain and record BP

Box 5
Indications for terminating exercise testing

Absolute indications
- Drop in systolic blood pressure of >10 mg Hg from baseline blood pressure despite an increase in workload, when accompanied by other evidence of ischemia
- Moderate to severe angina
- Increasing nervous system symptoms (eg, ataxia, dizziness, or near-syncope)
- Signs of poor perfusion (cyanosis or pallor)
- Technical difficulties in monitoring ECG or systolic blood pressure
- Subject's desire to stop
- Sustained ventricular tachycardia
- ST elevation ($\geq$1.0 mm) in leads without diagnostic Q-waves (other than V1 or aVR)

Relative indications
- Drop in systolic blood pressure of $\geq$10 mm Hg from baseline blood pressure despite an increase in workload, in the absence of other evidence of ischemia
- ST or QRS changes such as excessive ST depression (>2 mm of horizontal or downsloping ST-segment depression) or marked axis shift
- Arrhythmias other than sustained ventricular tachycardia, including multifocal PVCs, triplets of PVCs, supraventricular tachycardia, heart block, or bradyarrhythmias
- Fatigue, shortness of breath, wheezing, leg cramps, or claudication
- Development of bundle branch block or IVCD that cannot be distinguished from ventricular tachycardia
- Increasing chest pain
- Hypertensive response[a]

Abbreviations: ECG, electrocardiogram; ICD, implantable cardioverter-defibrillator discharge; IVCD, intraventricular conduction delay; PVCs, premature ventricular contractions. [a]In the absence of definitive evidence, the committee suggests systolic blood pressure of greater than 250 mm Hg and/or a diastolic blood pressure of greater than 115 mm Hg. Modified from Fletcher et al.

From Gibbons RJ, Balady GJ, Bricker JT, Chaitman BR, Fletcher GF, Froelicher VF, Mark DB, McCallister BD, Mooss AN, O'Reilly MG, Winters WL Jr. ACC/AHA 2002 guideline update for exercise testing: summary article: a report of the ACC/AHA Task Force on Practice Guidelines (Committee to Update the 1997 Exercise Testing Guidelines). J Am Coll Cardiol 2002;40:1531–40.

- Cool down
  - The patient may walk slowly on the treadmill before the belt is stopped completely
  - Duration of slow walk varies according to clinical preference
  - Prolonged slow walking may limit detection of recovery ST-segment depression[24]
  - Immediate supine position may be preferred to assure detection
- Continue patient monitoring for a minimum of 6 minutes in recovery
  - Print and review ECG every minute
  - Obtain BP reading every 1 to 2 minutes
  - Assess the patient for signs or symptoms of concern, including chest pain, lightheadedness, worsening dyspnea
- Criteria for terminating monitoring:
  - Any ECG changes have resolved to baseline level
  - BP has stabilized and is within 10 mm Hg of supine baseline
  - Pulse has stabilized and within reasonable range of baseline, typically less than 100 bpm
  - Any symptoms or signs occurring during exercise have resolved
  - Patient feeling subjectively "normal"

Interpretation of results

With completion of the testing protocol and recovery monitoring, a report of findings and conclusions should be documented. The interpretation of an exercise stress test considers both objective and subjective parameters and attempts to predict the likelihood of obstructive CAD and assess overall prognosis. This involves the evaluation of ECG findings, hemodynamic changes, patient-reported symptoms, and exercise capacity. The test may be ruled positive, negative, uninterpretable, or equivocal. Whether the test is positive or negative depends on the presence or absence of signs and symptoms indicative of myocardial ischemia. Uninterpretable tests tend to be due to factors preventing identification of inducible ischemia on ECG, such as left bundle branch block (LBBB) or significant artifact. A test may be deemed equivocal if the provider finds insufficient evidence to rule the test positive or negative, but there may be continued clinical concern.

Evidence of ischemia

ST changes should be read at 60 to 80 ms from the J point and any changes noted present in 3 consecutive beats.[21,25] ECG changes that may indicate myocardial ischemia include

- $\geq$2 mm rapidly upsloping ST depression where the slope is greater than 1 mV/s
- Greater than 1.5 mm slowly upsloping ST depression where slope is less than 1 mV/s (**Fig. 2**)
- $\geq$1 mm or more horizontal or downsloping ST depression (**Figs. 3** and **4**)[26]
- $\geq$1 mm ST elevation in patients without myocardial ischemia history and with a normal baseline[27]
- >1 mm of ST elevation in leads with baseline Q wave for patient with known prior myocardial ischemia[21]
- Normalization of resting ST-segment elevation or T-wave inversion with exercise (except young patients with resting early repolarization)[21]
- T-wave inversion in two or more contiguous leads without baseline Q waves

Ischemic ST-segment changes can also be seen during the recovery phase of the ECG stress test. ST-segment depression during recovery is associated with increased

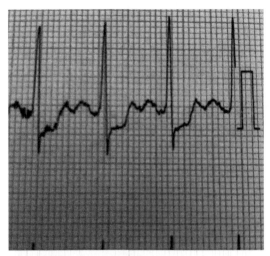

Fig. 2. Slowly upsloping ST-segment depression.

cardiovascular mortality in patients with and without known CAD.[28,29] ST changes in recovery have similar prognostic significance to ST changes that occur during stress testing and increase the test's sensitivity.[30,31]

Rhythm Response
While there are many normal rhythm variations that can occur during exercise,[9] some impact prognosis and require documentation in the interpretation report.

- Left bundle branch block—The incidence of exercise-induced LBBB is low (0.4%–1.1%[32]), and its significance in assessing CAD risk is unclear. Limited evidence from case reports suggests that exercise-induced LBBB is associated with a nearly 3-fold increased risk of death or major cardiac events,[27] while other

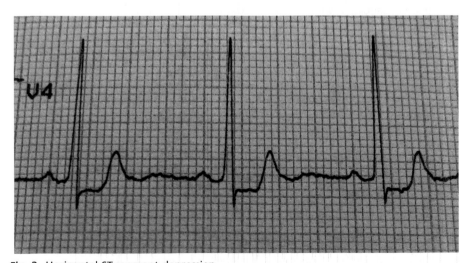

Fig. 3. Horizontal ST-segment depression.

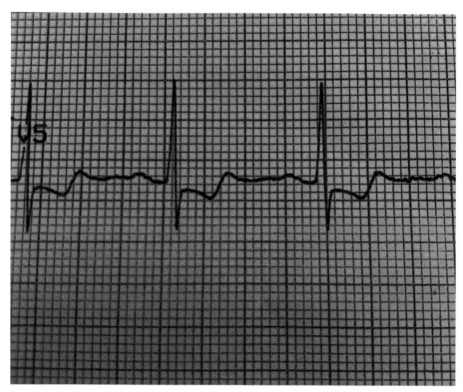

Fig. 4. Downsloping ST-segment depression.

reports suggest risk is only increased when associated with ischemic symptoms or other ECG changes.[33] ST-segment changes in the context of LBBB are non-diagnostic; however, ST segment changes that occur before the development of, or after the resolution of, exercise-induced LBBB may be interpreted as usual.[27]

- Ventricular arrhythmia—Ectopy from the ventricle is common during exercise and is associated with increasing age. Exercise-induced ventricular ectopy raises concern in those with cardiomyopathy, valvular heart disease, history of severe myocardial ischemia, and family history of sudden cardiac death. Patterns of ventricular ectopy and their significance vary widely. In general, increasing frequency and complexity of ectopy during exercise is associated with increased cardiac risk, especially when ectopy occurs in conjunction with other concerning ECG or hemodynamic changes.[21] In one study, patients with ventricular ectopy seen during the recovery phase had a 5-year all-cause mortality rate of 9% compared with 5% in those without recovery phase ectopy.[32] Any sustained ventricular tachycardia (>30 seconds duration) is highly concerning and is a criterion for test termination.[21]
- Supraventricular arrhythmias—Premature atrial contractions are seen in both healthy and diseased hearts during exercise. Atrial fibrillation and atrial flutter are rarely triggered by exercise. Advanced age, lung disease, alcohol, and caffeine have been identified triggers, but CAD is not commonly associated.[9]
- Atrioventricular (AV) blocks—Exercise induction of Mobitz type II and complete (third degree) AV blocks may be related to inducible ischemia. In both cases, the test should be stopped immediately.[9]

Heart rate response and recovery

In response to exercise, HR normally increases in a progressive manner. An inadequate HR response to exercise is termed chronotropic incompetence and linked to increased cardiac events and all-cause mortality.[9] In one study, for patients who achieved a workload of ≥10 Metabolic Equivalents, those reaching less than 85% of their MPHR were approximately four times more likely to have perfusion defects than those who reached greater than 85% of their MPHR.[11]

Heart rate recovery (HRR) is a useful variable when interpreting an ECG stress test.[34] Its definition has varied in both time and extent of decrease. A decrease of less than 12 beats per minute within the first minute of recovery is commonly considered abnormal.[35] Patients with an abnormal HRR were more likely to have perfusion defects (23% vs 19% in those with normal HRR) on thallium scintigraphy despite no differences in ST-segment change or angina during stress testing. Additionally, patients with an abnormal HRR were found to have higher 6-year mortality than those with normal HRR (19% vs 5%).[34]

Blood Pressure Response

BP changes during exercise ECG stress testing can help predict CAD. Systolic blood pressure (SBP) during exercise ≥210 mm Hg for men and ≥190 mm Hg for women is termed a hypertensive, or exaggerated, BP response and is associated with increased risk for future hypertension, left ventricular hypertrophy, and adverse cardiovascular events.[9] Additionally, an increase in diastolic blood pressure (DBP) during exercise of greater than 10 mm Hg from baseline or a DBP of ≥90 mm Hg is abnormal and also predicts increased risk of CAD.[9] SBP normally decreases by 15% in the first 3 minutes of recovery after exercise stress testing.[7] The ratio of SBP at 3 minutes into the recovery phase to the SBP at peak exercise is known as the SBP recovery ratio. The SBP recovery ratio is considered abnormal if it is greater than 0.9 and has similar diagnostic accuracy to ST segment depression for identifying CAD.[7,36] Similarly, exercise-induced hypotension, a decrease in SBP below its baseline value, is associated with an increased risk of adverse cardiovascular events and all-cause mortality.[37–39]

Functional capacity

Cardiovascular fitness can be quantified by calculating the total METS achieved during testing. One MET, or metabolic equivalent, is defined as the amount of oxygen consumed at rest and is equal to 3.5 mL O_2/kg/min.[40] The energy expenditure of the test is a multiple of the base MET. Measurement of METS during ECG stress test can help predict cardiovascular events. The higher the intensity that a patient can achieve during exercise, the higher their survival rate, regardless of their age or gender.[41] Patients who achieve a workload of 10 or more METS during an ECG stress test have more than a 5-fold decrease in prevalence of reversible ischemic defect and 2.6-fold decrease in fixed perfusion defects when compared with patients who achieve less than 7 METS. They also have a 17-fold decrease in the prevalence of significant ischemia, defined as greater than 10% of the left ventricle, compared with those achieving less than 7 METS.[8]

POSTTEST MANAGEMENT AND PROGNOSIS

If the patient has a positive ECG stress test, the patient should be considered for formal referral to cardiology for consideration of invasive angiography.[42] The ACC and AHA recommend coronary angiography be performed in high-risk posttest patients, further evaluation and individualized clinical judgment on intermediate-risk posttest patients, and observation and medical management in low-risk posttest patients.[42,43] One of multiple prognostic tools, the Duke Treadmill Score (DTS), can help provide prognostic information to providers by combining multiple factors into one measure.[7]

DTS = Exercise duration − (ST deviation × 5) − (Angina Index × 4)

- Exercise duration (in minutes)
- ST deviation (in mm),
- Angina index (none = 0, typical angina = 1, angina causing testing cessation = 2)

Scores of ≥5 are low risk and can be observed or medically managed; scores of ≤−11 are high risk and should be referred to cardiology for further management. Patients with intermediate risk should receive additional evaluation through MPI. The DTS does not account for other predictors of CAD such as ventricular ectopy, abnormal HRR, and SBP recovery. Patients with these findings should have further evaluation with advanced imaging or referral to cardiology based on the provider's clinical judgment. For patients with inconclusive tests (eg, inability to reach THR), additional testing with advanced imaging may improve diagnostic certainty.[44]

Activity recommendations can be derived from clinical and calculated assessments obtained through the exercise ECG stress test. Functional capacity, maximum HR achieved, and BP response can assist with guidance on lifestyle modifications and exercise recommendations. METS achieved can be correlated with specific activities of daily life and exercise and can inform a prescription of activity, intensity, and duration to help improve health and increase functional capacity.[45,46]

SUMMARY

For the primary care physician, chest pain is a common complaint with a broad differential diagnosis that requires attention to rule out life-threatening potential etiologies. Multiple diagnostic tools augment clinical evaluation and decision-making, each offering variable accuracy, availability, and cost. Evidence-based and consensus guidelines can inform the clinician's decision about whether office-based exercise ECG stress testing is an appropriate diagnostic test choice.

Exercise ECG stress testing is a well-studied, patient-centric, cost-efficient cardiac risk assessment tool that can be used in the primary care clinic. It allows the primary care physician to gather information for diagnosing CAD and estimating cardiovascular risk, as well as recommending treatment interventions, need for further testing, or referral to cardiology. Finally, exercise stress testing provides data that can be used in lifestyle modification and exercise recommendations.

CLINICS CARE POINTS

- Determining a patient's risk of CAD by evaluating quality of chest pain and estimating pretest probability are critical steps when deciding on the most appropriate stress testing modality.

- Baseline vitals and ECG should be obtained as part of preprocedural evaluation before testing to exclude contraindications to stress testing.

- Thorough patient education and instruction will facilitate procedure efficiency on testing day and increase patient comfort.

- The decision to stop medications, including beta-blockers, requires clinical evaluation of the risks and benefits of the medication.

- Target heart rate should not be used as the sole criterion for measuring adequate workload for terminating exercise stress testing.

- It is important to monitor for signs of inducible ischemia both during exercise and the recovery phase.
- Heart rate recovery is a valuable prognostic marker.

DISCLOSURE

The authors have nothing to disclose.

REFERENCES

1. Lozano R, Naghavi M, Foreman K, et al. Global and regional mortality from 235 causes of death for 20 age groups in 1990 and 2010: a systematic analysis for the Global Burden of Disease Study 2010. Lancet 2012;380(9859):2095–128.
2. Fihn SD, Gardin JM, Abrams J, et al. American College of Cardiology Foundation/ American Heart Association Task Force. 2012 ACCF/AHA/ACP/AATS/PCNA/ SCAI/STS guideline for the diagnosis and management of patients with stable ischemic heart disease: a report of the American College of Cardiology Foundation/American Heart Association task force on practice guidelines, and the American College of Physicians, American Association for Thoracic Surgery, Preventive Cardiovascular Nurses Association, Society for Cardiovascular Angiography and Interventions, and Society of Thoracic Surgeons. Circulation 2012; 126(25):e354–471.
3. Rosamond W, Flegal K, Furie K, et al. Heart disease and stroke statistics–2008 update: a report from the American Heart Association Statistics Committee and Stroke Statistics Subcommittee. Circulation 2008;117:e25–146.
4. Mozaffarian D, Benjamin EJ, Go AS, et al. Executive Summary: Heart Disease and Stroke Statistics–2016 Update: A Report From the American Heart Association. Circulation 2016;133:447–54.
5. Nichols M, Townsend N, Scarborough P, et al. Cardiovascular disease in Europe 2014: epidemiological update. Eur Heart J 2014;35(42):2950–9.
6. Garner KK, Pomeroy W, Arnold JJ. Exercise stress testing: indications and common questions. Am Fam Physician 2017;96(5):293–9.
7. Bourque JM, Beller GA. Value of Exercise ECG for Risk Stratification in Suspected or Known CAD in the Era of Advanced Imaging Technologies. JACC Cardiovasc Imaging 2015;8(11):1309–21.
8. Bourque JM, Holland BH, Watson DD, et al. Achieving an exercise workload of $\geq$10 METS predicts a very low risk of inducible ischemia: does myocardial perfusion imaging have a role? J Am Coll Cardiol 2009;54(6):538–45.
9. Fletcher GF, Ades PA, Kligfield P, et al. Exercise standards for testing and training: a scientific statement from the American Heart Association. Circulation 2013;128:873.
10. Sabharwal NK, Stoykova B, Taneja AK, et al. A randomized trial of exercise treadmill ECG versus stress SPECT myocardial perfusion imaging as an initial diagnostic strategy in stable patients with chest pain and suspected CAD: cost analysis. J Nucl Cardiol 2007;14(2):174–86.
11. Gianrossi R, Detrano R, Mulvihill D, et al. Exercise-induced ST depression in the diagnosis of coronary artery disease: A meta-analysis. Circ 1989;80(1):87–98.
12. Lee TH, Boucher CA. Clinical practice. Noninvasive tests in patients with stable coronary artery disease. N Engl J Med 2001;344(24):1840–5.
13. Gibbons RJ, Balady GJ, Bricker JT, et al. American College of Cardiology/American Heart Association Task Force on Practice Guidelines. Committee to Update the

1997 Exercise Testing Guidelines. ACC/AHA 2002 guideline update for exercise testing: summary article. A report of the American College of Cardiology/American Heart Association Task Force on Practice Guidelines (Committee to Update the 1997 Exercise Testing Guidelines). J Am Coll Cardiol 2002;40(8):1531–40.

14. Morise AP, Haddad WJ, Beckner D. Development and validation of a clinical score to estimate the probability of coronary artery disease in men and women presenting with suspected coronary disease. Am J Med 1997;102(4):350–6.

15. Pryor DB, Shaw L, McCants CB, et al. Value of the history and physical in identifying patients at increased risk for coronary artery disease. Ann Intern Med 1993;118(2):81–90.

16. Balady GJ, Arena R, Sietsema K, et al. Clinician's Guide to Cardiopulmonary Exercise Testing in Adults: A Scientific Statement From the American Heart Association. Circulation 2010;122(2):191–225.

17. Patel MR, Bailey SR, Bonow RO, et al. ACCF/SCAI/AATS/AHA/ASE/ASNC/HFSA/ HRS/SCCM/SCCT/SCMR/STS 2012 appropriate use criteria for diagnostic catheterization: a report of the American College of Cardiology Foundation Appropriate Use Criteria Task Force, Society for Cardiovascular Angiography and Interventions, American Association for Thoracic Surgery, American Heart Association, American Society of Echocardiography, American Society of Nuclear Cardiology, Heart Failure Society of America, Heart Rhythm Society, Society of Critical Care Medicine, Society of Cardiovascular Computed Tomography, Society for Cardiovascular Magnetic Resonance, and Society of Thoracic Surgeons. J Am Coll Cardiol 2012;59(22):1995–2027.

18. Herbert WG, Dubach P, Lehmann KG, et al. Effect of B-Blockade on the interpretation of the exercise ECG: ST level versus delta-STHR index. Am Heart J 1991;122(Iss 4, Pt 1):993–1000.

19. Myers J, Arena R, Franklin B, et al. Recommendations for Clinical Exercise Laboratories: A Scientific Statement from the American Heart Association. Circulation 2009;119(24):3144–61.

20. Rodgers GP, Ayanian JZ, Balady G, et al. American College of Cardiology/American Heart Association Clinical Competence statement on stress testing: a report of the American College of Cardiology/American Heart Association/American College of Physicians—American Society of Internal Medicine Task Force on Clinical Competence. J Am Coll Cardiol 2000;36(4):1441–53.

21. Clinical exercise testing and interpretation. In: Riebe D, Ehrman JR, Liguori G, et al, editors. ACSM's guidelines for exercise testing and prescription. 10th ed. Philadelphia: Wolters Kluwer; 2016. p. 111–42.

22. Borg GA. Psychophysical bases of perceived exertion. Med Sci Sports Exerc 1982;14(5):377–81.

23. Health-related physical fitness testing and interpretation. In: Riebe D, Ehrman JR, Liguori G, et al, editors. ACSM's guidelines for exercise testing and prescription. 10th ed. Philadelphia: Wolters Kluwer; 2016. p. 66–110.

24. Aggarwal SP, Wander GS, Bala K, et al. Effect of posture in immediate post-exercise period on ischaemic ST-changes during stress electrocardiographic testing. Indian Heart J 1994;46(6):307–9.

25. Kharabsheh SM, Al-Sugair A, Al-Buraiki J, et al. Overview of exercise stress testing. Ann Saudi Med 2006;26(1):1–6.

26. Rijneke RD, Ascoop CA, Talmon JL. Clinical significance of upsloping ST segments in exercise electrocardiography. Circulation 1980;61:671.

27. Vaidya GN. Application of exercise ECG stress test in the current high cost modern-era healthcare system. Indian Heart J 2017;69(4):551–5.

28. Aronow WS. Correlation of ischemic ST-segment depression on the resting electrocardiogram with new cardiac events in 1,106 patients over 62 years of age. Am J Cardiol 1989;64:232.
29. Miranda CP, Lehmann KG, Froelicher VF. Correlation between resting ST segment depression, exercise testing, coronary angiography, and long-term prognosis. Am Heart J 1991;122:1617.
30. Lachterman B, Lehmann KG, Abrahamson D, et al. "Recovery only" ST-segment depression and the predictive accuracy of the exercise test. Ann Intern Med 1990;112(1):11–6. Erratum in: Ann Intern Med 1990;113(4): 333-4.
31. Fearon WF, Lee DP, Froelicher VF. The effect of resting ST segment depression on the diagnostic characteristics of the exercise treadmill test. J Am Coll Cardiol 2000;35:1206.
32. Frolkis JP, Pothier CE, Blackstone EH, et al. Frequent ventricular ectopy after exercise as a predictor of death. N Engl J Med 2003;348(9):781–90.
33. Vasey C, ODonnell J, Morris S, et al. Exercise-induced left bundle branch block and its relation to coronary artery disease. Am J Cardiol 1985;56:892–5.
34. Cole CR, Blackstone EH, Pashkow FJ, et al. Heart-rate recovery immediately after exercise as a predictor of mortality. N Engl J Med 1999;341:1351–7.
35. Desai MY, De la Pena-Almaguer E, Mannting F. Abnormal heart rate recovery after exercise as a reflection of an abnormal chronotropic response. Am J Cardiol 2001;87:1164–9.
36. Tsuda M, Hatano K, Hayashi H, et al. Diagnostic value of postexercise systolic blood pressure response for detecting coronary artery disease in patients with or without hypertension. Am Heart J 1993;125:718–25.
37. Dubach P, Froelicher VF, Klein J, et al. Exercise-induced hypotension in a male population. Criteria, causes, and prognosis. Circulation 1988;78:1380–7.
38. Morris CK, Morrow K, Froelicher VF, et al. Prediction of cardiovascular death by means of clinical and exercise test variables in patients selected for cardiac catheterization. Am Heart J 1993;125:1717–26.
39. O'Neal WT, Qureshi WT, Blaha MJ, et al. Systolic Blood Pressure Response During Exercise Stress Testing: The Henry Ford Exercise Testing (FIT) Project. J Am Heart Assoc 2015;4(5):e002050.
40. Jetté M, Sidney K, Blümchen G. Metabolic equivalents (METS) in exercise testing, exercise prescription, and evaluation of functional capacity. Clin Cardiol 1990;13(8):555–65.
41. Myers J, Prakash M, Froelicher V, et al. Exercise capacity and mortality among men referred for exercise testing. N Engl J Med 2002;346(11):793–801.
42. Herner M, Agasthi P. Cardiac Stress Imaging. [Updated 2020 Oct 7]. In: StatPearls [Internet]. Treasure Island (FL): StatPearls Publishing; 2020. Available from: https://www.ncbi.nlm.nih.gov/books/NBK563161/.
43. Miller TD, Askew JW, Anavekar NS. Noninvasive Stress Testing for Coronary Artery Disease. Heart Fail Clin 2016;12(1):65–82.
44. Blankstein R, DeVore AD. Selecting a Noninvasive Imaging Study After an Inconclusive Exercise Test. Circulation 2010;122(15):1514–8.
45. Benefits and risks associated with physical activity. In: Riebe D, Ehrman JR, Liguori G, et al, editors. ACSM's guidelines for exercise testing and prescription. 10th ed. Philadelphia: Wolters Kluwer; 2016. p. 1–21..
46. Ainsworth BE, Haskell WL, Whitt MC, et al. Compendium of physical activities: an update of activities codes and MET intensities. Med Sci Sport Exerc 2000;32(9 Suppl):S498–516.

Performance and Interpretation of Office Spirometry

Jonathon Firnhaber, MD, MAEd, MBA

KEYWORDS

- Pulmonary function testing • Spirometry • Obstructive lung disease
- Restrictive lung disease

KEY POINTS

- Spirometry is easily accomplished in the primary care physician's office; evaluation of lung volumes and diffusion capacity—the additional components of pulmonary function testing—require advanced equipment and are typically performed in a pulmonary laboratory setting.
- Interpretation of spirometry involves both numerical flow and volume data and evaluation of the morphology of the flow-volume curve.
- Decreased flow relative to lung volume, reflected in the forced expiratory volume in the first second/forced vital capacity ratio, is the hallmark of obstructive lung disease.
- Reduced vital capacity, with relatively normal flow rates, is the hallmark of restrictive lung disease.
- Acceptability and reproducibility criteria for spirometry help ensure data are of sufficient quality to be clinically useful.

INTRODUCTION

Pulmonary function testing (PFT) is an important component of the evaluation, monitoring, and management of patients with dyspnea or established lung disease.

PFT can help the clinician answer several important questions:
1. Does this patient have lung disease? And is the disease of a significant degree that it may be responsible for a patient's presenting symptoms?
2. What is the predominant pattern of lung disease? Obstructive and restrictive patterns of disease each imply different pathophysiologic processes.
3. Is this patient's lung disease evolving over time? Serial pulmonary function tests are needed in this case.

Three evaluations fall under the umbrella of "pulmonary function tests":

Brody School of Medicine, East Carolina University, 101 Heart Drive, Greenville, NC 27834, USA
E-mail address: firnhaberj@ecu.edu

Prim Care Clin Office Pract 48 (2021) 645–654
https://doi.org/10.1016/j.pop.2021.07.004
0095-4543/21/© 2021 Elsevier Inc. All rights reserved.

primarycare.theclinics.com

1. Flow rates, evaluated with spirometry,
2. Lung volumes, and
3. Diffusion capacity.

Spirometry is easily accomplished in the primary care physician's office; evaluation of lung volumes and diffusion capacity requires advanced equipment and is typically performed in a pulmonary laboratory setting.

NATURE OF THE PROBLEM

Clinicians are relatively inaccurate at predicting both the severity of patients' airflow limitation and the nature of that limitation, leading to both under- and overdiagnosis of lung disease, including chronic obstructive pulmonary disease (COPD) and asthma.[1,2] Patients may minimize or accommodate to their symptoms and subsequently not recognize the importance of controller medications that may decrease their risk of complications and mortality. Spirometry can verify the presence of disease for a patient, thereby increasing motivation to pursue lifestyle changes and medication adherence. Spirometry alone may support, but does not establish, a diagnosis.

Multiple guidelines, including those published by the American Thoracic Society (ATS) and the European Respiratory Society (ERS),[3] the Global Initiative for Chronic Obstructive Lung Disease (GOLD),[4] and the National Asthma Education Program (NAEP)[5] recommend the use of spirometry or PFTs to correctly diagnose COPD and asthma. ATS/ERS, GOLD, and the US Preventive Services Task Force[6] recommend against using spirometry to screen asymptomatic adults for COPD. GOLD guidelines do, however, suggest that in individuals with symptoms or risk factors for COPD—such as greater than 20 pack-years of smoking or recurrent chest infections—the diagnostic yield of spirometry favors its use as a method of early case finding. Despite national and international guidelines recommending its use, spirometry is underutilized in the primary care setting.

INDICATIONS AND CONTRAINDICATIONS

ATS/ERS[5] outlines indications for spirometry:

- Diagnostic:
  - Evaluate symptoms, signs, or abnormal laboratory tests
  - Measure the effect of disease on pulmonary function
  - Screen individuals at risk of having pulmonary disease
  - Assess preoperative risk
  - Assess prognosis
  - Assess health status before beginning a strenuous physical activity program
- Monitoring:
  - To assess therapeutic intervention
  - To describe the course of diseases that affect lung function
  - For people exposed to injurious agent
  - For adverse reactions to drugs with known pulmonary toxicity
- Disability/impairment evaluations to assess
  - Patients as part of a rehabilitation program
  - Risks as part of an insurance evaluation
  - Individuals for legal reasons
- Public health:
  - Epidemiologic surveys
  - Derivation of reference equations

○ Clinical research

ATS/ERS[5] additionally outlines relative contraindications for spirometry to include conditions affected by

- Increases in myocardial demand or changes in blood pressure:
  ○ Acute myocardial infarction within 1 week
  ○ Systemic hypotension or severe hypertension
  ○ Significant atrial or ventricular arrhythmia
  ○ Noncompensated heart failure
  ○ Acute cor pulmonale
  ○ Clinically unstable pulmonary embolism
  ○ History of syncope related to forced expiration or cough
- Increases in intracranial or intraocular pressure:
  ○ Cerebral aneurysm
  ○ Brain surgery within 4 weeks
  ○ Recent concussion with continuing symptoms
  ○ Eye surgery within 1 week
- Increases in sinus and middle ear pressures:
  ○ Sinus surgery or middle ear surgery or infection within 1 week
- Increases in intrathoracic and intraabdominal pressure:
  ○ Presence of pneumothorax
  ○ Thoracic surgery within 4 weeks
  ○ Abdominal surgery within 4 weeks
  ○ Late-term pregnancy

Additional relative contraindications include active or suspected transmissible respiratory or systemic infection or condition predisposing to transmission of infection, such as hemoptysis, significant secretions, oral lesions, or oral bleeding.

PULMONARY FUNCTION TESTING

Variables measured during spirometry include

1. Forced vital capacity (FVC).
   - FVC is most commonly decreased in restrictive processes, although may also be decreased in more severe obstruction.
   - Vital capacity (VC) measured with a forced expiration may be less than when measured with a slower exhalation. In obstructive disease, such as asthma or COPD, forced expiration triggers premature closure of small airways and limits the total volume that is exhaled—termed "air trapping."
   - Older adults, particularly those with obstructive lung disease, may exhale more slowly and have difficulty maintaining the expiratory effort necessary to achieve FVC. FEV_6—forced expiratory volume in 6 seconds—is an acceptable alternative to FVC. FEV_6 offers equally useful data with a less physically demanding test.
2. Forced expiratory volume in the first second of the FVC maneuver (FEV_1).
   - The initial phase of exhalation is marked by airflow in large airways. As exhalation progresses, air flows from medium to progressively smaller airways.
   - FEV_1 primarily evaluates resistance to airflow in large- and medium-sized airways.
   - Both FEV_1 and FVC are reported in comparison to population-derived reference values matched for age, gender, height, and race.
3. Forced expiratory flow $(FEF)_{25-75}$, also termed "maximal midexpiratory flow."

- FEF_{25-75} measures the airflow during the middle one-half of expiration—from when 25% of FVC is exhaled until the point 75% of FVC is exhaled.
- FEF_{25-75} is more variable than FVC or FEV_1 and is primarily affected by small airways obstruction and disease.

Lung volumes can be quantified by 2 methods:

1. Dilution testing, where a known volume of inert gas, such as helium, is inhaled. The inhaled gas is diluted by gas already present in the lungs, and its concentration in exhaled gas reflects the initial volume of gas within the lungs.
2. Body plethysmography, where the patient sits in an airtight box and performs breathing maneuvers. Volume and pressure changes measured within the box allow calculation of lung volumes.

Lung volume testing measures functional residual capacity and VC directly and residual volume (RV) and total lung capacity (TLC) indirectly. Decreased TLC is characteristic of a restrictive process. Elevated TLC indicates hyperinflation and elevated RV indicates air trapping; this combination of findings is typically seen with obstructive lung disease.

Fig. 1 outlines clinically relevant lung volumes and capacities.

Diffusion capacity is typically measured using carbon monoxide and evaluates the rate of transfer of gas from the alveolus to hemoglobin. The available alveolar surface area, relative permeability of the alveolar-capillary membrane, and hemoglobin concentration can all affect the rate of gas diffusion. The primary diseases that affect each of these variables are

- Emphysema, which decreases available alveolar surface area, and
- Parenchymal lung disease, such as interstitial fibrosis, which decreases permeability of the alveolar-capillary membrane.

Intrapulmonary hemorrhage may increase measured diffusion capacity, as inhaled carbon monoxide is taken up by erythrocytes within the alveolar spaces.

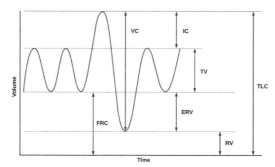

Fig. 1. Clinically relevant lung volumes and capacities. (1) Total lung capacity (TLC): total volume of gas within the lungs after maximal inspiration. (2) Residual volume (RV): volume of gas remaining in the lungs after maximal expiration. (3) Vital capacity (VC): volume of gas expired during maximal expiration—difference between TLC and RV. (4) Functional residual capacity (FRC): volume of gas remaining in the lungs in the resting state or after a tidal expiration. (5) Tidal volume (TV): volume of gas moved during resting (tidal) respiration. (6) Inspiratory capacity (IC): volume of gas moved between tidal expiration and maximal inspiration. (7) Inspiratory reserve volume (IRV): volume of gas moved between tidal and maximal inspiration. (8) Expiratory reserve volume (ERV): volume of gas moved between tidal and maximal expiration. (*Courtesy of* Michael Firnhaber, PhD, Boulder, CO.)

PROCEDURAL APPROACH
Equipments Needed for Office Spirometry

- Spirometer
  - Multiple manufacturers and models of spirometer are available for use in the office setting. It is important for the clinician to verify that their spirometer conforms to the standards established by ATS. Each manufacturer will provide its recommended cleaning and maintenance schedule.
  - The volume accuracy of the spirometer should be calibrated daily using a fixed volume (typically 3-L) syringe (**Fig. 2**).
- Nose clip
- Bronchodilator, such as albuterol metered dose inhaler (90 mcg per puff) or nebulized solution (0.083%: 2.5 mg per 3 mL)
- A private room helps to minimize distractions from the testing procedure.

Performing the Spirometry Test

- A brief history is obtained, including smoking history, current medications, recent illness, and current symptoms.
- The clinician should confirm that the patient has not engaged in any activities that may affect their ability to perform the test or may alter the results of the test, including
  - Smoking or vaping within 1 hour
  - Consuming intoxicants within 8 hours
  - Performing vigorous exercise within 1 hour
  - Wearing clothing that restricts full chest and abdominal expansion[5]
- The patient's weight and height (without shoes) should be recorded; these values are used to determine predicted normal values for FEV_1 and FVC.
- The test procedure is explained to the patient, emphasizing the importance of following directions and giving best effort. It may be helpful for the technician performing the test to demonstrate an appropriate testing exhalation.
- The patient is seated upright, with head slightly elevated and a nose clip in place (**Fig. 3**).
- At the end of a tidal exhalation, the patient closes his/her lips around the spirometer mouthpiece.
- The patient inhales fully and rapidly to TLC.

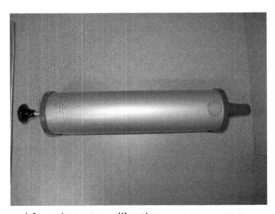

Fig. 2. 3-L syringe used for spirometer calibration.

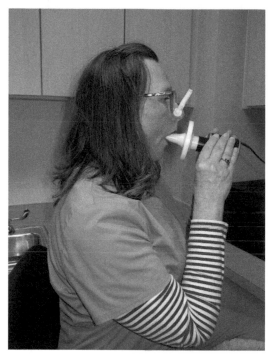

Fig. 3. Patient demonstrating correct positioning, use of nose clip, and placement of spirometer mouthpiece during testing.

- ○ Some spirometry machines do not record an inspiratory curve. If that is the case, the patient can close his/her lips around the spirometer mouthpiece immediately following full inhalation.
- After minimal (<1 second) pause, the patient exhales rapidly and fully until he/she is not able to exhale any further. The patient should start the exhalation with a forceful "blast" rather than a gradual increase in expiratory flow. It is important for the technician performing the test to loudly and enthusiastically coach the patient to continue to exhale ("blow, blow, keep going, blow, blow!") until the patient is unable to expel any more air and the low point of VC is reached. Testing software with visual cues to continue to exhale can supplement the technician's encouragement.
- The patient is allowed to recover, and the maneuver is repeated a minimum of 3 times or until reproducibility of the examination is verified.
- If postbronchodilator testing is requested, a short-acting bronchodilator is administered. Testing is paused for 15 to 20 minutes to allow the medication to have its full effect, then the testing process is repeated.
- If at any point the patient complains of dizziness or lightheadedness, the testing procedure may be paused or terminated if symptoms persist. Forceful exhalation substantially increases intrathoracic pressure, which decreases venous return to the heart and transiently decreases cardiac output.

Acceptability and Reproducibility Criteria

- The spirometry testing procedure is not inherently simple. There are multiple points where artifact may be introduced into the data, and inconsistent patient effort may result in considerable variability between tests.

- ATS has established acceptability and reproducibility criteria for spirometry that help ensure data are of sufficient quality to be clinically useful.
- Most spirometry software will guide the technician to continue the testing sequence until acceptability and reproducibility criteria are met.
- Acceptability criteria include spirograms that are
  - Free from artifact, such as cough and air leak
  - Have good starts
  - Have satisfactory exhalation, with smooth, continuous, and maximal effort and at least 6 second duration or a plateau in the volume-time curve
- Reproducibility criteria include 3 spirograms with FEV_1 and FVC with less than 0.15 L of variance between tests.
  - If reproducibility criteria have not been met after 8 tests have been performed, or if the patient is unable to continue testing, the testing is terminated.

INTERPRETATION

Interpretation of spirometry involves evaluation of numerical flow and volume data and the flow-volume curve morphology. Flow rates and volumes are measured with the spirometer, as the patient forcibly and completely exhales after a maximal inspiration. Maximal forced expiration describes VC or TLC minus RV.

The graphic portion of a spirometry report is the flow-volume loop (or the flow-volume curve If It Includes only the expiratory portion). Various disease processes trigger characteristic changes in the morphology of the flow-volume loop.

Although each clinician may have a preferred sequence for evaluating spirometry data, a consistent stepwise approach is most important. The potential approaches include the following:

1. Evaluate vital capacity
   - FVC is expressed as a percentage of predicted value.
   - Reduced vital capacity, with relatively normal flow rates, is the hallmark of restrictive lung disease. Restrictive lung disease is a heterogenous group of disorders, broadly grouped into pleural, alveolar, interstitial, neuromuscular, and thoracic cage abnormalities.
   - Reduced VC may be seen in obstructive lung disease, particularly when significant air trapping is present. In this case, the degree of severity of both flow rate reduction and vital capacity will be roughly equivalent.
   - *FVC*
     80%–120% of predicted value: Normal
     70%–79%: Mild reduction
     50%–69%: Moderate reduction
     <50%: Severe reduction
2. Evaluate flow rates.
   - FEV_1, expressed as a percentage of predicted value, is a helpful data point but is more useful when expressed as a percentage of FVC: FEV_1/FVC or $FEV_1\%$.
   - Decreased flow relative to lung volume, reflected in the FEV_1/FVC ratio, is the hallmark of obstructive lung disease.
   - *FEV_1/FVC*
     >75%–80%: Normal
     60%–75%: Mild obstruction
     50%–59%: Moderate obstruction
     <50%: Severe obstruction

- Note: different guidelines recommend different ranges for characterizing severity of obstruction; there is no universally accepted set of ranges.
- Although FEF_{25-75} is not included in formal spirometry interpretation algorithms, many clinicians recognize the variable as an indicator of small airway obstruction. FEF_{25-75} may be decreased before changes in FEV_1 are apparent, particularly in smokers, and this can be indicated on a spirometry interpretation as "decreased FEF_{25-75} suggests early small airways disease."

3. Characterize pattern of abnormality, if any.

	Normal	Obstruction	Restriction	Mixed
FEV_1/FVC	Normal	Reduced	Normal	Reduced
FVC	Normal	Normal	Reduced	Reduced

The appearance of the flow-volume loop offers additional insight into the underlying disease process; its pattern is at least as important as the flow and volume data (**Fig. 4**).

- With increasing degrees of obstruction, the flow-volume curve (expiratory loop) becomes progressively more "scooped out" or concave when compared with a normal curve. Midflow obstruction, demonstrated by a decrease in $FEF_{25-75,}$ contributes to the concave appearance of the flow-volume curve and may be apparent before FEV_1 is significantly decreased. As obstruction becomes more severe, the height of the curve, representing peak expiratory flow rate, decreases and the "tail" of the curve may lengthen as well.
- With increasing degrees of restriction, the flow-volume curve (expiratory loop) becomes progressively more vertical and narrower, with loss of the "tail" of a normal curve.

4. Evaluate reversibility, if any.
- Bronchodilator reversibility in adults is defined as an increase in FEV_1 of greater than or equal to 12% and ≥ 200 mL from baseline; in children, an increase in FEV_1 of $\geq 12\%$ alone demonstrates reversibility.
- Obstructive defects associated with asthma will typically show complete or near-complete reversibility in postbronchodilator testing.
- Obstructive defects associated with COPD will typically show minimal or no reversibility in postbronchodilator testing. A significant proportion of patients with COPD have some degree of airway hyperreactivity and may, therefore, demonstrate a positive response to bronchodilator.
- Improvement in FVC postbronchodilator, using the same greater than 12% increase and greater than 200 mL criteria, suggests the prebronchodilator decrease in FVC was due to an obstructive process.

5. Evaluate need for additional pulmonary testing.
- Patients with a restrictive pattern, or a mixed pattern with no demonstrated postbronchodilator reversibility, should be referred for full PFTs including lung volumes and diffusion capacity.
- Patients with a clinical history of asthma, but normal spirometry, may be candidates for bronchoprovocation testing. Various inhaled agents may be used, including methacholine, histamine, and mannitol. Methacholine challenge has a high negative predictive value and can be helpful to rule out asthma.[7] This testing is more commonly performed in a pulmonary laboratory setting.

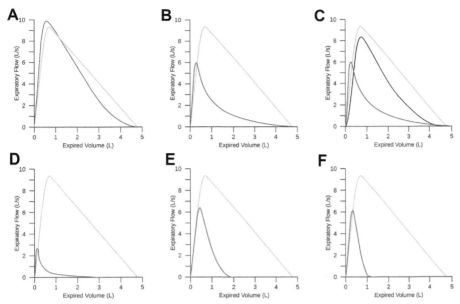

Fig. 4. Common patterns of flow-volume curves and associated disease processes. (*A*) Normal. Some deviation from the predicted curve (*gray line*) is expected, but the general shape of the flow-volume curve is consistent across patients with normal lung function. (*B*) Moderate obstruction. The height of the curve—peak expiratory flow rate (PEFR)—is decreased and the midportion of the curve is "coved" or "scooped out" with a flattened tail at the end of exhalation. (*C*) Moderate obstruction with reversibility. The prebronchodilator curve (*blue line*) depicts moderate obstruction; the postbronchodilator curve (*red line*) more closely approximates a normal or predicted pattern. (*D*) Severe obstruction. The height of the curve (PEFR) is markedly decreased and abruptly transitions to a long, flat tail of minimal flow. (*E*) Moderate restriction. The PEFR is decreased with a shortened tail, corresponding to decreased total expired volume. (*F*) Severe restriction. The flow-volume curve is narrow, with an abrupt decline in flow and no tail. (*Courtesy of* Michael Firnhaber, PhD, Boulder, CO.)

CLINICS CARE POINTS

- Accurate measurement of patient height and weight is critical in the determination of predicted values for spirometrically measured variables.
- The quality of data obtained during spirometry hinges on the patient's ability to follow directions and put forth their best effort; enthusiastic coaching can augment patient motivation.
- Spirometry alone may support, but does not establish, a diagnosis; patient history, physical findings, and imaging studies augment the data obtained with PFT.
- The appearance of the flow-volume loop offers additional insight into the underlying disease process; its pattern is at least as important as the flow and volume data.

DISCLOSURE

The author has nothing to disclose.

REFERENCES

1. Diab N, Gershon AS, Sin DD, et al. Under-diagnosis and Over-diagnosis of Chronic Obstructive Pulmonary Disease. Am J Resp Crit Care 2018;198(9):1130–9.
2. Aaron SD, Boulet LP, Reddel HK, et al. Underdiagnosis and Overdiagnosis of Asthma. Am J Resp Crit Care 2018;198(8):1012–20.
3. Halpin DMG, Criner GJ, Papi A, et al. Global Initiative for the Diagnosis, Management, and Prevention of Chronic Obstructive Lung Disease. The 2020 GOLD Science Committee Report on COVID-19 and Chronic Obstructive Pulmonary Disease. Am J Resp Crit Care 2021;203(1):24–36.
4. National Heart, Lung and Blood Institute. Expert Panel Report 3 (EPR3): guidelines for the diagnosis and management of asthma. Bethesda (MD): NHLBI; 2007.
5. Graham BL, Steenbruggen I, Miller MR, et al. Standardization of Spirometry 2019 Update. An Official American Thoracic Society and European Respiratory Society Technical Statement. Am J Resp Crit Care 2019;200(8):e70–88.
6. Siu AL, Bibbins-Domingo K, Gillman M, et al. Screening for Chronic Obstructive Pulmonary Disease: US Preventive Services Task Force Recommendation Statement. JAMA 2016;315(13):1372–7.
7. Cockcroft DW. Direct Challenge Tests Airway Hyperresponsiveness in Asthma: Its Measurement and Clinical Significance. Chest 2010;138(2):18S–24S.

ADDITIONAL REFERENCES

Dempsey TM, Scanlon PD. Pulmonary Function Tests for the Generalist: A Brief Review. Mayo Clin Proc 2018;93(6):763–71.

Godfrey MS, Jankowich MD. The Vital Capacity Is Vital Epidemiology and Clinical Significance of the Restrictive Spirometry Pattern. Chest 2016;149(1):238–51.

Hankinson JL, Eschenbacher B, Townsend M, et al. Use of forced vital capacity and forced expiratory volume in 1 second quality criteria for determining a valid test. Eur Respir J 2015;45(5):1283–92.

King-Biggs MB. Asthma. Ann Intern Med 2019;171(7):ITC49.

Kjellberg S, Houltz BK, Zetterström O, et al. Clinical characteristics of adult asthma associated with small airway dysfunction. Resp Med 2016;117:92–102.

Krol K, Morgan MA, Khurana S. Pulmonary Function Testing and Cardiopulmonary Exercise Testing An Overview. Med Clin North Am 2019;103(3):565–76.

Langan RC, Goodbred AJ. Office Spirometry: Indications and Interpretation. Am Fam Physician 2020;101(6):362–8.

Parker MJ. Interpreting spirometry: the basics. Otolaryngol Clin North Am 2014;47(1):39–53.

Ruppel GL, Enright PL. Pulmonary Function Testing. Respir Care 2012;57(1):165–75.

Primary Care Removal of Fishhooks, Rings, and Foreign Bodies from the Ear, Nose, and Superficial Eye and Conjunctiva

J. Lane Wilson, MD*

KEYWORDS

- Nasal foreign body • Aural foreign body • External auditory canal foreign body
- Superficial eye foreign body • Corneal abrasion • Corneal epithelial injury
- Fishhook removal • Ring removal

KEY POINTS

- Unless lodged near a vital structure, most embedded fishhooks can safely be removed in the office using one of several commonly described techniques.
- Entrapped rings on digits without signs of ischemia or associated deformity can often be removed in the office with noncutting techniques or a hand cutter.
- Embedded earrings of the earlobe may be removed in the office with a cooperative patient.
- Foreign bodies of the external auditory canal may be removed in the office via irrigation or with one of several commonly used office surgical tools chosen based on the foreign body size, shape, and composition.
- Clinicians may make multiple attempts using positive pressure techniques or one or 2 attempts to remove intranasal foreign bodies with one of several commonly used office surgical tools chosen based on the foreign body size, shape, and composition.
- Recently acquired, small, superficial, and noninfected corneal or conjunctival foreign bodies can often be removed in the office.

 Video content accompanies this article at http://www.primarycare.theclinics.com.

Department of Family Medicine, East Carolina University Brody School of Medicine, 101 Heart Drive, Greenville, NC 27834, USA
* Corresponding author.
E-mail address: wilsonjo@ecu.edu

Prim Care Clin Office Pract 48 (2021) 655–676
https://doi.org/10.1016/j.pop.2021.07.005
0095-4543/21/© 2021 Elsevier Inc. All rights reserved.

INTRODUCTION

Embedded fishhooks, digital ring entrapment, and foreign bodies of the ear, nose, and superficial eye and conjunctiva commonly present to emergency departments and urgent care offices, but they also present to primary care clinics. Many of these conditions can be managed in the primary care office. In this guide, effective, pragmatic, and safe techniques for removal of the offending objects are reviewed specifically for the primary care office setting.

FISHHOOK REMOVAL
Background

Recreational fishing is the second most reported outdoor recreational activity by Americans and is popular worldwide.[1] Injuries with fishhooks (**Fig. 1**) are common, and most are relatively superficial. Many embedded hooks are removed in the field and never present to care. Because of the trajectory of a hook attached to a line, the point is generally pulled in a trajectory parallel to it, thus preventing deep penetration. However, hook injuries may also occur via other mechanisms that could lead to deeper penetrating injuries, such as when baiting, removing a hook from a caught fish, grabbing an unseen hook, or stepping on a lure.

When evaluating a patient who has presented to care with an embedded hook, a quick history should focus on the mechanism of injury, the type of hook involved, and what attempts at removal before arrival had taken place. Tetanus status should also be ascertained. Physical examination should focus on the depth of injury, the type of tissue involved, and whether there is any neurovascular compromise or bone involvement.

Techniques

Five main techniques have been described in the literature. Comparative data on techniques are limited because the method selected for removal depends on the location

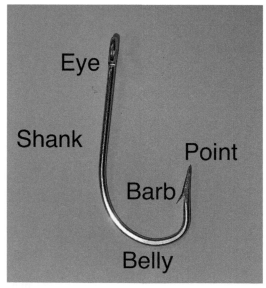

Fig. 1. Anatomy of a fishhook.

of the penetrating trauma, the depth of the trauma, and the type of hook.[2] In general, atraumatic methods (back-out, string-yank) are attempted before any technique that introduces additional trauma (needle cover, advance and cut). Finally, the cut-it-out technique is used as a last resort after failure of other methods.[3–5] The back-out technique is primarily reserved for barbless hooks or injuries in which the barb is not embedded. The other techniques focus on the neutralization of the barb to facilitate removal.

Before hook removal, any line, bait, lures, or other items attached to the hook should be removed. If a treble hook or other hook with multiple points is embedded (**Fig. 2**), the free points should be cut below the barb or taped to prevent secondary injuries. Local cleaning of the wound and hook with povidone iodine or chlorhexidine should be performed before attempted removal. For particularly dirty wounds, irrigation with saline may be helpful.

The back-out and string-yank techniques often do not require the administration of local anesthesia; however, if other techniques are required, the hook is embedded deeply, or patient cooperation would limit the ability to perform the removal safely, local anesthesia is advised.[5] If there is concern for nerve injury, sensory examination should be performed before administration of local anesthetic. Because fingers are often sites of injury, digital blocks are frequently used.

Back-Out or Retrograde Technique

Hooks without barbs are easily removed using the back-out technique and have the advantage of causing minimal or no additional trauma. In this technique, after prepping the skin, the shank of the hook is grasped with hemostats and backed out along

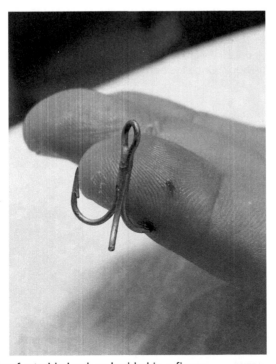

Fig. 2. An example of a treble hook embedded in a finger.

the track of the hook. Given the speed, ease, and atraumatic nature of this technique, local anesthesia is not often required and may in fact be more painful than more prompt removal of the hook.

If attempted in a superficially embedded barbed hook, downward pressure should be applied to the shank in an attempt to disengage the barb before backing out along the path of the embedded hook. If any resistance is met with this effort, this technique should be abandoned in favor of one of the subsequently described techniques.[3–5]

String-Yank or String Technique

The string-yank method is highly successful and often used in the field. Multiple commercial products that use the principles of this technique are available, and advice on how to perform the technique is readily available online in fishing magazines, blogs, and video channels. Like with the back-out technique, local anesthesia is often not required but should be considered. This technique has the advantages of being easy to perform, quick, relatively atraumatic, and highly successful. This technique should not be attempted on hooks embedded in earlobes or other nonfixed tissue.

First, a string or silk suture should be wrapped or tied around the belly of the hook. One hand should grasp the loose ends of the string in an orientation to provide tension parallel to the shank. The other hand is then used to provide a perpendicular downward pressure on the shank in an effort to disengage the barb from tissue and move it into the path of injury. Once this downward pressure has been applied, a sharp, forceful jerk or yank should be applied to the string (**Fig. 3**, Video 1). The practitioner and others in the room should wear eye protection and be mindful of the expected trajectory of the hook.[3–5]

Needle Cover or Needle Technique

A large-bore needle is used to cover and provide an exit pathway for the barb in the needle cover technique. After local wound care and administration of anesthetic along the path of injury, an 18-gauge or larger needle is advanced parallel to the shank along the embedded hook until the barb is covered. To do so, the bevel of the needle should face the inside of the hook. Once the barb is covered, the hook and needle are backed

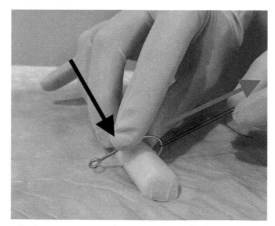

Fig. 3. String yank technique. Downward pressure is applied perpendicularly to the shank of the hook (*black arrow*) while the other hand jerks or yanks the string in a direction parallel to the shank (*blue arrow*).

out as a single unit. The needle cover technique is the most technically difficult method to perform and is best used for large hooks that are superficially embedded.[3-5]

Advance and Cut or Push-Through Technique

In the advance and cut technique, the shank is grasped with hemostats or needle drivers and the hook is advanced along the curve of the belly to create an exit wound through which the barb is exposed. Local anesthesia should therefore cover the area through which the hook is advanced. Once the barb is exposed, it is cut off with wire cutters. The remaining hook is the removed via the retrograde technique.

An alternative to cutting the barb off and backing the remaining hook out is the advance without cut method. In this method, the eye of the hook is cut off and the hook is advanced in its entirety through the created exit wound. This method may be preferable to advance and cut if there are multiple barbs (termed baitholder hooks) on the shank of the hook.

There are certain situations in which advancing the hook is not possible, like if a fingernail, vital structure, or bone would obstruct the point's path through, and other techniques must be considered.[3-5]

Cut-It-Out Technique

This technique is sometimes described as an alternative way to perform the needle cover technique. As it is the most invasive measure with the potential to introduce further tissue trauma, it is generally reserved if other attempts at removal have been unsuccessful.

To perform, a number 11 scalpel blade is advanced parallel to the shank along the pathway of injury analogous to the needle pathway in the needle cover technique. Once the incision reaches the barb, the hook is removed via the now expanded traumatic pathway. If the hook is deeply embedded and a clear exit pathway is still not possible after the scalpel incision reaches the barb, blunt dissection may be indicated to expand the opening in an effort to minimize further soft tissue trauma.[3-5]

Special Considerations

Fishhooks lodged in or near the orbit, eyelid, urethra, testicle, or superficial major vessels, such as the carotid artery, warrant subspecialty surgical consultation before attempted removal.

Aftercare

In most cases, fishhook wounds should be allowed to heal by secondary intention, regardless of the technique used for removal. Once the hook is removed, the wound should be explored for foreign bodies and irrigated. Topical antibiotic ointment and a simple dressing is then applied. Tetanus prophylaxis should also be given when indicated.

Systemic antibiotics generally are not indicated, and there are no studies evaluating their use for prophylaxis. Antibiotics may be considered in certain cases, however. Any injury involving tendon, cartilage, or bone is associated with a high risk for infection. Similarly, immunocompromised patients and those with conditions resulting in poor wound healing warrant consideration for prophylactic antibiotics. When antibiotics are given for prophylaxis, they should be directed toward skin flora and those organisms that typically cause cellulitis.[3-5]

RING REMOVAL
Background

Rings may become entrapped over a digit (most often finger) when an incorrectly sized ring is forced on or when a digit becomes swollen distal to a correctly sized ring. Penile rings are usually placed for sexual purposes and become entrapped after subsequent swelling. Entrapped penile rings should be removed with consultation from urology, and therefore specific techniques and procedures are not reviewed in this discussion.

The history should focus on the reason for the digital swelling. Common causes are trauma, allergic reaction (local or systemic), infection (most commonly cellulitis), weight gain, and medical conditions that may cause generalized edema. In most cases, patients have already tried various methods to remove the ring without success.

The physical examination is most important to identify signs of ischemia. Mottling or discoloration, severe pain, loss or significant delay of capillary refill, and absence of pulse-by-pulse oximetry are indications of ischemia and should prompt emergent removal. Emergent removal is also indicated if there is an associated open wound or deformity[6] (**Box 1**).

Techniques

The technique chosen depends on 2 factors: whether there is need for emergent removal and the composition of the ring (**Fig. 4**).[6–12] Before any of the noncutting procedures, elevation and icing of the finger can be done in an effort to reduce swelling. Anesthesia using a digital block is usually necessary. An advantage of avoiding a digital block before a cutting procedure is the ability of the patient to give feedback if the ring overheats during the procedure. Digits should be prepped with povidone iodine or chlorhexidine before removal procedures.

Manual Removal Techniques

After elevation, application of ice, and lubrication, the ring may be able to be removed manually. One method of removal involves applying dorsal pressure to the ring while advancing the ventral aspect. Once advanced, pressure is applied on the ventral aspect and the dorsal aspect is advanced. This procedure is known as the caterpillar technique.[7]

Two other methods of manual removal have been described that first involve compressive reduction of distal finger edema. In the double Penrose drain method, one Penrose drain is wrapped just distal to the proximal interphalangeal joint and serves as a tourniquet. A second Penrose drain is then wrapped tightly from the tourniquet proximally until it reaches the ring. Once the edema has been sufficiently reduced, the ring is advanced past the proximal interphalangeal joint and the first Penrose drain is removed.[8]

Box 1
Indications for emergent consultation with hand, plastic, or orthopedic surgeon

Signs of ischemia
Digital nerve injury
Associated deep wound, fracture, joint dislocation, or tendinous injury
For penile ring entrapment, emergency urologic consultation is indicated

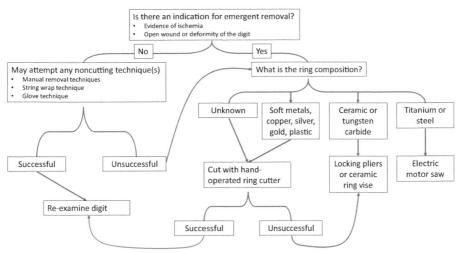

Fig. 4. Algorithm for entrapped ring removal. Data from Refs.[6-12]

A second compressive method involves tightly wrapping the finger from the tip proximally to the ring with a Penrose drain or other material, such as elastic wrap or tape. The extremity is then raised above the heart for 10 to 15 minutes. A blood pressure cuff may be used as a tourniquet before removal of the compressive material to prevent recurrence of edema during removal attempts.[9]

String Pull

Various methods have been described using a loop or loops of string to advance an entrapped ring. After lubricating the digit, a string, suture, or elastic band is passed under the ring and pulled through such that the 2 ends are even and easily grasped together. Traction is then applied to the string distally and moved in a circular fashion to advance a small portion of the ring at a time. Additional strings may be added to prevent slippage or loss of progress as the ring advances or to provide more circumferential traction on the ring.[10]

An alternative is to hold 2 strings parallel along the sides of the digit by an assistant to provide gentle traction. The practitioner then performs the alternating pressure and advancement of the dorsal and volar aspects of the digit as in the caterpillar technique.[11]

String Wrap

First, a string, umbilical tape, Penrose drain, suture, or dental floss is passed under the ring from the distal side to the proximal side. The proximal end of the string is secured to the palm or wrist with tape. Beginning at the distal edge of the ring, the string is tightly wrapped, working to cover all tissue while progressing distally until the proximal interphalangeal joint is traversed. Once compression is complete, the proximal end of the string is pulled on distally. As it unwraps around the finger, the ring will advance until it passes the proximal interphalangeal (PIP) joint, at which point it will generally pass freely **(Fig. 5**, Video 2).[6]

Glove Technique

The glove technique is similar to some of the string techniques but allows for circumferential traction along the ring in its entirety. To perform, a finger is cut from a surgical

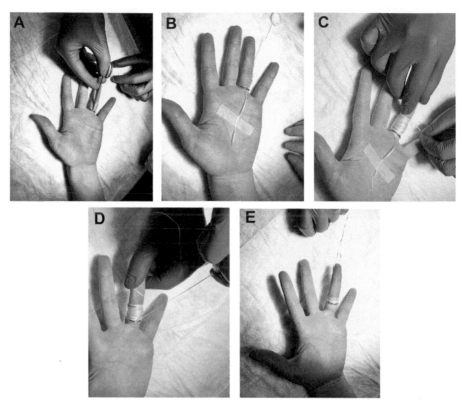

Fig. 5. String wrap technique. (*A*) The string is passed under the ring from the distal to the proximal side. (*B*) The string is secured to the palm with tape. (*C*) The string is wrapped tightly around the finger from the distal end of the ring working distally past the proximal interphalangeal joint. (*D,E*) The proximal end of the string is pulled distally, causing it to unwrap and advance the ring.[6]

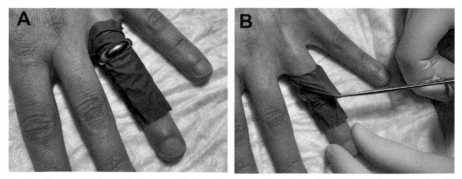

Fig. 6. Glove technique. (*A*) A cutoff glove finger is placed on the affected finger under the entrapped ring. (*B*) The portion of the glove proximal to the ring is then inverted and traction is applied distally to advance the ring.[12]

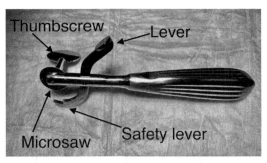

Fig. 7. Hand ring cutter.

glove at the base and again at the tip to form a tube; this is slid over the affected finger, and the proximal end is passed under the ring using mosquito forceps or other small-caliber tool. A lubricant is applied to the glove. The portion of the glove proximal to the ring is then inverted and traction is applied distally to advance the ring (**Fig. 6**).[12]

Ring Cutters

If there is an indication for emergent removal or the noncutting technique attempts fail, the ring should be cut. The type of device used depends on the composition of the ring.

For plastic or soft metal rings (eg, gold, silver, copper), a hand cutter may be used (**Fig. 7**). To perform, the safety lever is slipped under the ring and the lever is depressed to secure the ring in place and bring the serrated saw down upon it (**Fig. 8**). The thumbscrew is then turned manually to cut. After making a complete cut, it may be necessary to make a second cut to remove the ring. Metal filings left behind can be rinsed away with saline irrigation.

For harder metals, pliers found in many emergency departments can be effective. Although hard and difficult to cut, pincers can shatter tungsten carbide rings when pressure is applied. Finally, electric hand saws, Dremel saws, diamond-tipped saws, and dental drills are options when other methods have failed.[6] These tools are generally not available in primary care offices. High-speed cutting tools can

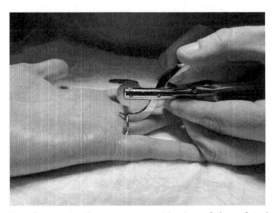

Fig. 8. Hand ring cutter demonstrating proper positioning of the safety lever under the ring before depressing the lever to bring the serrated saw down upon it.

generate considerable heat, and care must be taken to avoid burning the patient's skin while cutting.

Aftercare

Digits should be reexamined following ring removal for evidence of trauma, wound contamination, tendon function, and neurovascular compromise. Any finding of ischemia, fracture, or tendinous injury should prompt hand surgery consultation. Tetanus status should be assessed for any patient with trauma and contaminated wounds.

FOREIGN BODIES OF THE PINNA
Background

Embedded earrings represent the vast majority of foreign bodies of the pinna; this is most commonly found in young girls who do not practice appropriate self-care. Most cases involve the earlobe, but they can occur in the tragus or other cartilaginous areas of the outer ear. Complicating infection may be present in over a third of patients.[13]

Identification of the embedded earring is generally easy with palpation of the area. If pain limits this examination, plain films can confirm the presence of the earrings.

Contraindications to Primary Care Office Removal

Embedded piercings involving the cartilaginous portions of the ear are at high risk for chrondritis, perichondritis, and cartilage necrosis with resulting deformity and should be referred to otolaryngology for removal.[14]

Because most cases of embedded earrings occur in young children, some patients are unable to cooperate enough to safely perform the procedure without sedation and should be referred to otolaryngology.

Technique

The site should be prepped with povidone iodine or chlorhexidine and local anesthesia applied. The particular method of removal is similar in all circumstances but depends on which portion or portions of the earring are embedded:

- If the post and clip is embedded but the front of the earring is visible, posterior pressure should be applied to bring the backing or clip into view. Once in view, the post should be grasped with mosquito forceps, the backing removed, and then the front is easily removed. If the posterior pressure does not allow visualization of the backing or clip, a small incision on the posterior aspect of the earlobe can be made and the backing is bluntly dissected out.
- If the anterior portion of the earring is embedded but the backing or clip is visible, anterior pressure should be applied in an effort to bring the front of the earring into view. When in view, the post is clamped just behind the earring, the backing is removed, and then the front is removed. If unable to visualize the front earring with anterior pressure, a small incision can be made at the posterior piercing site and the front portion of the earring bluntly dissected out of the posterior piercing site.
- If neither the front nor the backing or clip is visible, a small incision is made on over the backing on the posterior earlobe and then the entire earring is bluntly dissected out as mentioned earlier.

Box 2
Indications for urgent otolaryngology referral before removal attempt

Button battery
Any evidence of injury to the EAC, TM, or middle ear
Penetrating foreign bodies (even if no evidence of existing penetrating
  injury)
Severe pain
EAC, external auditory canal; TM, tympanic membrane

Complications

Infection is a complicating factor in more than one-third of cases. Antibiotic coverage should be directed to cover methicillin-resistant *Staphylococcus aureus* and *Pseudomonas aeruginosa*. If abscess, chondritis, or perichondritis are suspected, parenteral antibiotics with the same spectrum of coverage should be initiated and otolaryngology consulted.[13,14]

Aftercare

Patients should be treated with topical antibiotic ointment, and the incision should be allowed to heal by secondary intention. Parents should be advised to delay repiercing of the ears until the child is old enough and motivated to practice sufficient self-care.[15]

FOREIGN BODIES OF THE EXTERNAL AUDITORY CANAL
Background

Most foreign bodies of the external auditory canal (EAC) are found in young children but may present in adults with cognitive impairments.[16,17] Most patients are asymptomatic, and the most common presentation is due to a parent or caregiver witnessing or suspecting placement of an object in the ear. When the objects do cause symptoms, ear pain, decreased hearing, and, rarely, otorrhea or cough or hiccups may occur.[18] Patients with live insects in the EAC may feel and hear it crawling, and it may be painful.

Otoscopy should be performed to assess the size, shape, and type of foreign body present. Beads and other spherical objects have the lowest success rates of removal.[17] The contralateral ear and nares should be examined for accompanying foreign bodies. **Boxes 2** and **3** list the indications for otolaryngology referral.

Contraindications

Irrigation is contraindicated in any patient with tympanic membrane (TM) perforation or tympanostomy tubes. Irrigation for organic matter foreign bodies should be used with

---

Box 3
Indications for elective otolaryngology referral

Glass or other sharp-edged foreign body
Any foreign body tightly wedged in the medial EAC
Any foreign body up against the TM with evidence of TM injury
Inability of patient to cooperate
EAC, external auditory canal; TM, tympanic membrane

---

great caution, because the material may absorb water, swell, and thus worsen obstruction. Button battery-related tissue necrosis can be worsened by the instillation of fluid and should be referred immediately to otolaryngology. Because spherical objects have such low rates of successful removal, elective referral to otolaryngology should be considered before removal attempt. **Boxes 2** and **3** detail the indications for otolaryngology referral.

Techniques

Irrigation

For small, nonorganic foreign bodies, or insects, irrigation is well tolerated and does not require direct visualization. Before performing, TM perforation and/or the presence of tympanostomy tubes should be excluded. Live insects should first be killed with the instillation of mineral oil or lidocaine.[19] In the author's experience, instilling a peroxide solution in the ear will often cause a live insect to crawl out of the canal within seconds, although this may result in an action-packed few seconds as everyone in the room reacts.

Patients are placed either in the supine position with the affected ear up, seated, or reclined. A towel or basin or other device to catch the irrigation solution is placed beneath the affected ear (**Fig. 9**). A 20- to 50-mL syringe loaded with tap water or saline is attached to plastic tubing (butterfly needle tubing or 14- to 16- gauge plastic intravenous catheter). The tubing is then directed to the superior and posterior aspect of the EAC and the plunger quickly depressed, thus allowing the solution to exit inferiorly and not interfere with the incoming stream. Multiple attempts may be necessary, or the object may move to a position better suited for instrumentation. This same technique may be used for impacted cerumen removal.

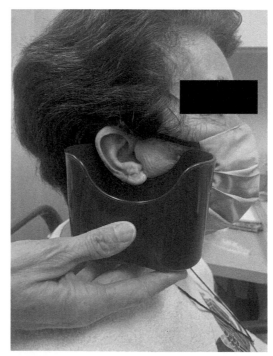

Fig. 9. Patient positioned for external auditory canal irrigation.

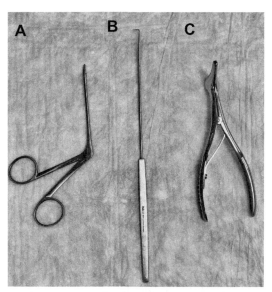

Fig. 10. Commonly used instruments for foreign body removal. (*A*) Alligator forceps, (*B*) right-angle hook, and (*C*) nasal speculum.

Instrumentation

Any removal attempt should be performed under direct visualization, and an operating head otoscope or headlight is essential. The EAC is sensitive and the procedure is likely to be painful, so caution should be exercised in any pediatric patient before attempting removal without appropriate restraint. This process is often not possible in the primary care setting, and a low threshold for referral to an otolaryngologist should be used.[17,20] Choosing an instrument (**Fig. 10**) for removal depends largely on the size, shape, and consistency of the foreign body:

- Soft, compressible foreign bodies or irregularly shaped objects or insects may be grasped with alligator forceps or other small surgical grasping tools.
- Smooth, solid objects are difficult to grasp and could be pushed further into the EAC if grasping it is attempted. A right-angle hook can be advanced to slip the point past the object, rotate the instrument, and then withdraw with the foreign body. This procedure carries risk for injury if the patient moves. Alternative tools using the same technique include angled cerumen curettes and angled wire loops.[16]
- In older and cooperative patients who can hold very still, cyanoacrylate glue may be applied to the end of a hollow plastic swab and adhered to the object. It takes at least 60 seconds for the glue to fully dry. Care must be taken to not push the object back further when applying pressure as the glue dries. Glue stuck to skin can be removed with 3% hydrogen peroxide or acetone.[21]

Techniques possible but not often available in primary care offices:

- Suction catheters may be applied to a smooth, round object.

Complications

Abrasion or laceration to the EAC is a common complication of foreign body removal and should be treated with topical antibiotic ear drops.

TM and middle ear injury are possible but rare. The risk can be minimized by following appropriate referral recommendations.

Complication rates increase with the number of attempts at foreign body removal.[17]

INTRANASAL FOREIGN BODY REMOVAL
Background

Intranasal foreign bodies most often occur in young children but may also present in adults with cognitive impairment. Often, they can go unnoticed for a long time due to lack of symptoms. The most common presentation is known history of foreign body without symptoms. When symptomatic, patients present with unilateral purulent discharge, foul odor, nasal obstruction or mouth breathing, and/or epistaxis.[22–24] Delay in diagnosis can lead to complications that include sinusitis, otitis media, periorbital cellulitis, and, rarely, meningitis.[25]

Indications

All intranasal foreign bodies should be removed. In the primary care setting, any nasal foreign body that is visible with a nasal speculum and without specific contraindication (see later discussion) can undergo multiple positive pressure attempts at removal and/or one or 2 attempts with instrumentation.[24]

Contraindications

Box 4 summarizes contraindications to primary care office removal of a nasal foreign body. In addition, inability to remove any object after 1 or 2 attempts should be followed by referral to an otolaryngologist.[24]

Techniques

Positive pressure techniques
Many nasal foreign bodies can be removed without instrumentation, particularly if they are smooth and totally occlusive. These techniques have the advantage of being able to be performed multiple times and are safe. Several methods have been described:

- The simplest method for children who are old enough to follow directions is to have the child occlude the unaffected naris and forcefully blow his or her nose.
- With the "parent's kiss" technique, the parent places his or her mouth entirely over the mouth of the child and occludes the unaffected naris. After slowly blowing air into the mouth of the child until some resistance is felt (indicating closure of the child's glottis), a forceful puff of air is given. This technique is effective in up to 60% of cases.[26]

Box 4
Indications for urgent otolaryngology referral before removal attempt

Button battery
Paired disk magnets
Posterior location unable to be easily visualized
Impacted foreign bodies with associated inflammation or infection
Penetrating foreign bodies (even if no evidence of existing penetrating
   injury)
Uncooperative patient prohibiting safe removal attempt in office

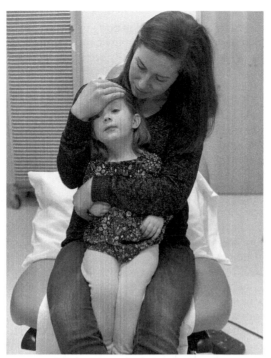

Fig. 11. Example of parent restraining a child in proper position for attempted intranasal foreign body removal: the child should sit on the parent's lap, legs restrained between the parent's thighs or under the parent's crossed legs, arms restrained by a parent's arm, and the head tipped back slightly and immobilized by the parent's other arm.

- As an alternative to the parent giving the puff of air by mouth-to-mouth contact, a straw may be used to administer the puff of air.
- A bag-valve mask may be used to complete the same procedures as the "parent's kiss."

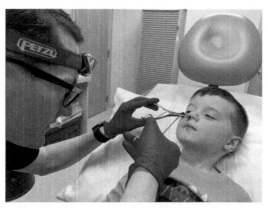

Fig. 12. Example of patient positioning for intranasal foreign body removal when parental restraint is not needed. A headlamp and nasal speculum are essential tools for adequate visualization.

Instrumental techniques

Before any attempt to remove a nasal foreign body by the practitioner, positioning and restraint of the child is paramount. Most primary care offices do not have restraint devices; however, many children can successfully be restrained by a parent for the short time it takes to make 1 or 2 attempts at removal. The child should sit on the parent's lap, legs restrained between the parent's thighs or under the parent's crossed legs, arms restrained by a parent's arm, and the head tipped back slightly and immobilized by the parent's other arm (**Fig. 11**). A headlight and nasal speculum should be used for examination (**Fig. 12**). Before removal attempt, a nasal decongestant spray and topical anesthetic should be administered.[24]

Choosing an instrument (see **Fig. 10**) for removal depends largely on the size, shape, and consistency of the foreign body:

- Soft, compressible foreign bodies may be grasped with alligator forceps, nasal packing forceps, or other small surgical grasping tools.
- Smooth, solid objects are difficult to grasp and could be pushed further into the nasal passage if this is attempted. A right-angle hook is advanced to slip the point past the object, the instrument is rotated, and then it is withdrawn with the foreign body. This procedure carries risk for injury if the patient moves. Alternative tools that use the same basic technique include ring curettes, wax loops, and bent paper clips.[27,28]
- In older and cooperative patients who can hold very still, cyanoacrylate glue may be applied to the end of a hollow plastic swab and adhered to the object. It takes at least 60 seconds for the glue to fully dry. Care must be taken to not push the object back further when applying pressure as the glue dries. Glue stuck to skin can be removed with 3% hydrogen peroxide or acetone.[21,28]

Techniques possible but not often available in primary care offices:

- Round, smooth objects may be removed with balloon catheters. Katz extractors are catheters specifically made for this purpose. The tip of the catheter is advanced past the object, the balloon is inflated (1 mL), and the catheter is withdrawn. This procedure often requires some topical anesthesia and lubrication to get the catheter tip past the object.
- Suction catheters may be applied to a smooth, round object.[27,28]
- A strong magnetic device may be used for some metallic objects.[28,29]

Special considerations

Button batteries necessitate immediate removal by an otolaryngologist due to the risk for alkaline tissue necrosis. Paired magnets on either side of the nasal septum can eventually lead to septal perforation from chronic compression.[21–23]

Complications

The most common complication of nasal foreign body removal is epistaxis after instrumentation. Epistaxis generally resolves with simple pressure.[21–23,25]

If a nasal foreign body goes undiagnosed for a prolonged time, sinusitis may be a presenting symptom and should be treated with antibiotics following removal of the object. There are rare reports of meningitis as a complication.[24]

Button batteries may cause alkaline tissue necrosis, and paired disk magnets may cause septal perforation.[21–23,25]

Aftercare
Unless treatment of a complication is required, no specific aftercare is usually indicated following nasal foreign body extraction.

SUPERFICIAL EYE FOREIGN BODY REMOVAL AND CORNEAL ABRASION
Background

Foreign bodies in the eye have often resulted in a corneal abrasion (also known as corneal epithelial defect) by the time of presentation, and, conversely, any presentation of a corneal abrasion should lead to investigation for the presence of a foreign body or foreign bodies. Therefore, foreign body removal and fluorescein examination are discussed in this section together.

Patients with foreign bodies of the eye or conjunctiva present with foreign body sensation, eye pain, red eye, persistent unilateral tearing, and/or known presence or suspicion of a foreign body. Those with corneal abrasion without foreign body present similarly but may have a different inciting event (eg, fingernail scratching the eye). History should focus on when the problem began, what the patient was doing when symptoms began, whether eye protection was being used, whether the patient wears contact lenses, and whether any potential high-velocity foreign bodies could be present. Contact lens wearers are at risk for spontaneous abrasions, particularly if habitually wearing the lenses longer than recommended or not following other routine hygiene measures.[30,31]

Examination of the eye should be performed with the goal of ruling out penetrating globe injury, traumatic hyphema, and infections. A small high-velocity foreign body can notably penetrate the globe without obvious symptoms or signs on examination. When possible, initial examination should be performed without topical analgesia. If pain prevents adequate examination, a single drop of a topical anesthetic may be used after penetrating globe injury is excluded with quick penlight examination (**Fig. 13**). Visual acuity testing should also be performed before any administration of topical anesthetic or fluorescein if possible.[31]

If the patient is unable to open the eye due to discomfort, the upper lid should be lifted and gently everted without the application of pressure onto the globe. A cotton-tip applicator may be used to achieve full eversion (**Fig. 14**). The lower lid can generally be everted with simple downward traction applied to the skin inferior to the lid over the zygoma (see **Fig. 13**).[32]

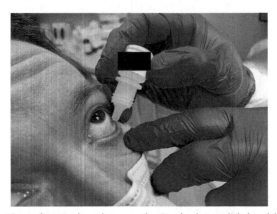

Fig. 13. Administration of topical ocular anesthesia: the lower lid should be retracted with one hand, the patient should be asked to look up, and 1 drop of anesthetic should be applied to the fornix.

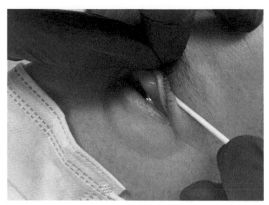

Fig. 14. Eversion of the upper lid using a cotton-tip applicator.

Fundoscopy should be performed to confirm a red reflex and evaluate for hyphema and hypopyon. Extraocular movement testing should not cause diplopia or significant increase in pain.

Indications

Patients presenting with a red eye, foreign body sensation, excessive unilateral tearing, exposure to UV light without protection (from tanning beds, welding machines, sunlight), mild trauma without concern for globe injury, hypersensitivity to light, or recent foreign body are candidates for fluorescein examination to evaluate for corneal epithelial injury.

Recently acquired, small, superficial, and noninfected corneal or conjunctival foreign bodies can often be removed in the office.[30,31]

Contraindications

Penetrating globe injuries and high-velocity injuries in which penetrating trauma could be difficult to detect are contraindications to fluorescein eye examination. An unknown chemical or known caustic chemical exposure can and should be irrigated, but no fluorescein examination should be attempted. The same contraindications apply to foreign body removal. In addition, foreign body removal should not be attempted in the primary care office if there is coexisting infection, ulceration, deeply embedded foreign bodies, or foreign bodies that have been present for more than 24 hours. Any contraindication to these procedures is cause for immediate ophthalmology referral.[30,31]

Techniques

Topical ocular anesthesia

After examination excludes globe penetration, the patient should be made to look upward, the lower lid should be retracted, and one drop of topical ocular anesthetic, such as 0.5% proparacaine or tetracaine solution, should be added into the lower fornix of the eye (see **Fig. 13**). The patient should have relief of pain within seconds of administration. For prolonged irrigation, this may need to be repeated every 5 to 10 minutes.

Corneal or Conjunctival Foreign Body Removal

Superficial corneal foreign bodies can often be removed via irrigation, especially if multiple small particulate materials are present. This process is easily achieved with warmed sterile saline solution in a syringe. The stream should not be aimed directly at the foreign body or cornea and should not be applied forcefully. If foreign bodies are present under the lid, eversion of the affected lid should be performed before irrigation.[30,31]

If irrigation is unsuccessful, removal under direct visualization with a moistened cotton-tipped swab can be attempted if the foreign body is superficial and small. Although irrigation can sometimes be performed without topical anesthesia, any attempt to remove a foreign body with a swab should be preceded by anesthetic administration. The patient should be placed in a comfortable position, usually supine, that stabilizes the head. The patient should be instructed to fix his or her gaze on a single point throughout the procedure. One hand should be anchored on the patient's zygoma, nasal bridge, or forehead as it is used to evert or retract the affected lid as applicable to the foreign body location. Alternatively, an assistant can assist with this portion of the procedure. With the other hand also anchored, the moistened cotton-tipped swab is used in a gentle rolling motion to lift the foreign body off the cornea. Direct pressure over the foreign body should not be applied. If the foreign body is not easily removed with this method, referral to an ophthalmologist is indicated.[30,31]

Fluorescein examination

If not performed before foreign body removal, fluorescein eye examination should strongly be considered following the procedure. If performed before foreign body removal, reexamination is indicated to evaluate for iatrogenic epithelial injury.

To administer, a single drop of saline or topical anesthetic should be first applied to the tip of a fluorescein strip. The lower lid of the patient is pulled downward like when administering topical anesthesia. The fluorescein strip is then either gently brushed against the exposed conjunctiva or a drop of liquid is allowed to fall into the fornix (Video 3). Blinking then distributes the stain quickly. A Wood lamp or the cobalt blue filter on a standard ophthalmoscope can then be used to examine for stained corneal defects.[30,31]

Common patterns of fluorescein staining are shown in **Fig. 14**. Foreign bodies may have a circumscribed stain around their edges. Conjunctival foreign bodies may cause a characteristic linear pattern in the upper eye caused by repetitive trauma from blinking.

Special Considerations

Pediatric patients

Pediatric patients may be more difficult to examine and often cannot provide a reliable history. Limited cooperation may necessitate administration of topical anesthesia before visual acuity examination. Some investigators recommend sweeping the conjunctiva for foreign bodies routinely. Management is otherwise similar to that of adults.[30,31]

Rust ring

Foreign bodies that contain iron may leave behind a rust ring. In the past, it has been common practice to remove these. However, routine removal carries risk of further damage and scarring, and most small rust rings will be resorbed over the course of a few days. If the corneal epithelium has not healed 2 to 3 days following the foreign body removal, referral to an ophthalmologist for debridement of the rust ring is indicated.[32]

Contact lenses

P aeruginosa is frequently a colonizer in contact lens wearers and places them at risk for superinfection of a corneal abrasion. Therefore, topical antibiotic selection for these patients should include those with antipseudomonal activity. Contact lenses should not be worn again until the abrasion and any comorbid infection is totally resolved.

Aftercare

Topical antibiotic ointments or drops should be considered in most patients with corneal abrasion. There is a notable lack of evidence for patient-oriented outcomes regarding antibiotic treatment. However, given the low-risk nature of topical antibiotics and the potential severe consequences of infection, expert opinion and anecdotal evidence suggests a low threshold to prescribe them.[30,31,33]

Ointments are typically preferable to drops because of their lubricating properties, which may facilitate epithelial healing. For non–contact lens-wearing patients, erythromycin 0.5% or sulfacetamide 10% ophthalmic ointments may be prescribed. If a patient would rather use drops, polymyxin/trimethoprim, sulfacetamide, or ciprofloxacin ophthalmic solutions are acceptable. For contact lens-wearing patients, antipseudomonal coverage with a topical fluoroquinolone ointment or drop is indicated.

Most corneal abrasions will heal overnight or within 48 hours. Duration of antibiotic therapy is thus based on expert opinion and practice experience given this fact. Patients may be instructed to use the antibiotics for 3 to 5 days, or, alternatively, 24 hours beyond resolution of symptoms. Any patient with symptoms persisting beyond 3 days should be referred to an ophthalmologist.[30,31]

Ophthalmologic solutions that contain steroids are contraindicated due to impairment of healing and risk for infection. Home topical anesthesia should also be avoided due to concern for delayed healing and potential to mask a more serious injury or complication. For the patient requesting analgesia, oral acetaminophen or nonsteroidal anti-inflammatory drugs (NSAIDs) are appropriate. Ophthalmic topical NSAID solutions are available but have the drawbacks of weak evidence of efficacy, expense, and pain on application.[34]

Patching is not recommended for routine practice and is contraindicated in patients with recent contact lens wear. Meta-analyses have demonstrated slowed healing, increased pain from the patch itself, and risk of injury due to loss of depth perception with patching. For certain cases with large abrasions, an ophthalmologist may apply a pressure patch.[35]

CLINICS CARE POINTS

- When removing embedded fishhooks, atraumatic removal techniques should be attempted before performing the cut-it-out technique.
- Entrapped rings without emergent indications for removal can often be removed intact using manual, compressive, string, or glove techniques.
- One attempt at removal of an EAC foreign body in the primary clinic office is appropriate if it is not a button battery, if there is existing evidence or significant risk of damaging the canal or TM, and if appropriate instrumentation is available for the size, shape, and consistency of the object.

- Multiple positive pressure technique attempts and one instrumentation attempt at intranasal foreign body removal in the primary care office is appropriate if it is not a button battery, paired disk magnets, or penetrating or potentially penetrating; it can be visualized with a nasal speculum; and if the appropriate instrumentation is available for the size, shape, and consistency of the object.

- Patients who present with foreign body sensation, eye pain, red eye, persistent unilateral tearing, and/or known presence or suspicion of a foreign body should be examined for the presence of a foreign body and corneal epithelial injury (corneal abrasion).

SUPPLEMENTARY DATA

Supplementary data to this article can be found online at https://doi.org/10.1016/j.pop.2021.07.005

DISCLOSURE STATEMENT

The author has nothing to disclose.

REFERENCES

1. Available at: https://www.statista.com/statistics/190202/number-of-participants-in-outdoor-activities-in-the-us-2009/. Accessed January 21, 2021.
2. Doser C, Cooper WL, Ediger WM, et al. Fishhook injuries: a prospective evaluation. Am J Emerg Med 1991;9:413–5.
3. Gammons MG, Jackson E. Fishhook removal. Am Fam Physician 2001;63(11): 2231–6.
4. Beasley K, Ouellette L, Bush C, et al. Experience with various techniques for fishhook removal in the emergency department. Am J Emerg Med 2019;37(5): 979–80.
5. Prats M, O'Connell M, Wellock A, et al. Fishhook removal: case reports and a review of the literature. J Emerg Med 2013;44(6):e375–80.
6. Kalkan A, Kose O, Tas M, et al. Review of techniques for the removal of trapped rings on fingers with a proposed new algorithm. Am J Emerg Med 2013;31(11): 1605–11.
7. Laurent St, Carla MD. The Caterpillar Technique for Removal of a Tight Ring. Anesth Analg 2006;103(4):1060–1.
8. Chiu TF, Chu SJ, Chen SG, et al. Use of a Penrose drain to remove an entrapped ring from a finger under emergent conditions. Am J Emerg Med 2007;25(6): 722–3.
9. Cresap CR. Removal of a hardened steel ring from an extremely swollen finger. Am J Emerg Med 1995;13(3):318–20.
10. Boe C, Kakar S. A Modified String Technique for Atraumatic Ring Removal. J Emerg Med 2018;55(2):240–3.
11. Burbridge MT, Ritter SE. An alternative method to remove a ring from an edematous finger. Am J Emerg Med 2009;27(9):1165–6.
12. Inoue S, Akazawa S, Fukuda H, et al. Another simple method for ring removal. Anesthesiology 1995;83(5):1133–4.
13. Timm N, Iyer S. Embedded earrings in children. Pediatr Emerg Care 2008; 24(1):31–3.
14. Fernandez AP, Neto IC, Anias CR, et al. Post-piercing perichondritis. Braz J Otorhinolaryngol 2008;74(6):933–7.

15. Fijałkowska M, Pisera P, Kasielska A, et al. Should we say NO to body piercing in children? Complications after ear piercing in children. Int J Dermatol 2011;50(4): 467–9.
16. Ansley JF, Cunningham MJ. Treatment of aural foreign bodies in children. Pediatrics 1998;101(4 Pt 1):638–41.
17. Karimnejad K, Nelson EJ, Rohde RL, et al. External Auditory Canal Foreign Body Extraction Outcomes. Ann Otol Rhinol Laryngol 2017;126(11):755–61.
18. Lossos IS, Breuer R. A rare case of hiccups. N Engl J Med 1988;318(11):711–2.
19. Leffler S, Cheney P, Tandberg D. Chemical immobilization and killing of intra-aural roaches: an in vitro comparative study. Ann Emerg Med 1993;22(12):1795–8.
20. Olajuyin O, Olatunya OS. Aural foreign body extraction in children: a double-edged sword. Pan Afr Med J 2015;20:186.
21. Persaud R. A novel approach to the removal of superglue from the ear. J Laryngol Otol 2001;115(11):901–2.
22. Hira İ, Tofar M, Bayram A, et al. Childhood Nasal Foreign Bodies: Analysis of 1724 Cases. Turk Arch Otorhinolaryngol 2019;57(4):187–90.
23. Morris S, Osborne MS, McDermott AL. Will children ever learn? Removal of nasal and aural foreign bodies: a study of hospital episode statistics. Ann R Coll Surg Engl 2018;100(8):1–3.
24. Ng TT, Nasserallah M. The art of removing nasal foreign bodies. Open Access Emerg Med 2017;9:107–12.
25. van der Veen J, Thorne S. Bacterial meningitis: a rare complication of an unrecognised nasal foreign body in a child. BMJ Case Rep 2017;2017. bcr2015209577.
26. Cook S, Burton M, Glasziou P. Efficacy and safety of the "mother's kiss" technique: a systematic review of case reports and case series. CMAJ 2012; 184(17):E904–12.
27. Schuldt T, Großmann W, Weiss NM, et al. Aural and nasal foreign bodies in children - Epidemiology and correlation with hyperkinetic disorders, developmental disorders and congenital malformations. Int J Pediatr Otorhinolaryngol 2019; 118:165–9. https://doi.org/10.1016/j.ijporl.2019.01.006.
28. Ng T-T. 20 ways of removing a nasal foreign body in the emergency department. Otorhinolaryngol Head Neck Sur 2016. https://doi.org/10.15761/OHNS.1000102.
29. Yeh B, Roberson JR. Nasal magnetic foreign body: a sticky topic. J Emerg Med 2012;43(2):319–21.
30. Wipperman JL, Dorsch JN. Evaluation and management of corneal abrasions. Am Fam Physician 2013;87(2):114–20.
31. Fraenkel A, Lee LR, Lee GA. Managing corneal foreign bodies in office-based general practice. Aust Fam Physician 2017;46:89.
32. Camodeca AJ, Anderson EP. Corneal Foreign Body. In: StatPearls [Internet]. Treasure Island (FL): StatPearls Publishing; 2020.
33. King JW, Brison RJ. Do topical antibiotics help corneal epithelial trauma? Can Fam Physician 1993;39:2349–52.
34. Wakai A, Lawrenson JG, Lawrenson AL, et al. Topical non-steroidal anti-inflammatory drugs for analgesia in traumatic corneal abrasions. Cochrane Database Syst Rev 2017;5:CD009781.
35. Lim CH, Turner A, Lim BX. Patching for corneal abrasion. Cochrane Database Syst Rev 2016;7:CD004764.

Office Management of Genitourinary and Gastrointestinal Procedures

Jonathon Firnhaber, MD, MAEd, MBA*, Bridgid Hast Wilson, MD, PhD

KEYWORDS

- Foley catheter insertion • Urinary catheter insertion • Suprapubic catheter exchange
- Thrombosed external hemorrhoid

KEY POINTS

- Urinary catheter insertion can be performed safely in outpatient primary care settings to relieve acute urinary obstruction.
- Exchange of suprapubic catheters can be performed in outpatient primary care settings for those patients with established stomas.
- Excision of thrombosed external hemorrhoids within the first 72 hours from the onset of symptoms offers improved clinical outcomes. After that time, spontaneous resolution may be better tolerated.

URINARY CATHETER PLACEMENT

Introduction

Urinary catheterization involves placing a tube through the urethra into the bladder lumen to drain urine. When a urinary catheter is needed for continued bladder drainage (indwelling) it is anchored within the bladder by filling a small balloon that surrounds the tube with saline. Most indwelling urinary catheters have 2 lumens, one channel to drain the bladder and one channel to inflate and deflate the anchoring balloon. Another type of catheter, a triple lumen catheter, has a third channel to allow for procedures such as continuous bladder irrigation or instillation of other solutions within the bladder, but this catheter type has limited use in the outpatient setting.

Indications for Urinary Catheterization

Acute urinary conditions that warrant urinary catheterization in the outpatient setting include urinary retention secondary to bladder outlet obstruction, benign prostatic hyperplasia, medication-induced retention, as well as evaluation for urinary tract infection in patients unable to spontaneously void. Chronic conditions are typically

Brody School of Medicine, East Carolina University, 101 Heart Drive, Greenville, NC 27834, USA
* Corresponding author.
E-mail address: firnhaberj@ecu.edu

Prim Care Clin Office Pract 48 (2021) 677–684
https://doi.org/10.1016/j.pop.2021.07.006
0095-4543/21/© 2021 Elsevier Inc. All rights reserved.

primarycare.theclinics.com

related to neurogenic bladder secondary to spinal cord injury, parkinsonism, or cerebral palsy. Although an indwelling catheter may be a temporary solution for neurogenic bladder, it should be noted that chronic bladder drainage may be better managed by a suprapubic catheter (SPC).

Anatomy

Planning for and insertion of a urinary catheter varies depending on the patient's sex due to urethral anatomy. The male urethra is long and has multiple anatomically distinct sections that may complicate insertion. Once the catheter is inserted into the urethral meatus, it must traverse the navicular fossa, penile urethra, bulbar urethra, membranous urethra, and finally the prostatic urethra before entering the bladder. The male urethra follows an "S-shaped" curve from the bulbar urethra through the membranous urethra and prostatic urethra that can cause some difficulty with catheter insertion.[1] In addition, any enlargement of the prostate can cause narrowing of the prostatic urethra resulting in an inability to pass the urinary catheter through it. Use of a Coude catheter, which has a firm upsloping tip, can help traverse a narrow prostatic urethra and other strictures.[1,2] The female urethra is relatively short in length and does not traverse anatomic structures that may complicate insertion. Pelvic organ prolapse and obesity may alter the external female anatomy making visualization of the urethra more challenging. Similarly, in postmenopausal women atrophy from decreased estrogen may make the urethral meatus take an anterior position that may obscure visualization.[1] Urethral strictures can occur in both males and females, particularly in patients who have had prior genitourinary surgeries or instrumentation. Inflammation from infection, trauma, or instrumentation can also compromise urethral integrity and make urethral injury more likely.

Preprocedure Planning

The diameter of a urinary catheter is measured on a French gauge where each French is equal to 0.33 mm. A 12F to 16F catheter is appropriate for most adult patients. If enlargement of the prostate or complications in traversing the prostatic urethra are expected, selection of a larger size, such as a 20F to 22F, may be prudent because this size has less risk of bending when encountering resistance.[2] A Coude catheter may also be used both for resistance at the prostatic urethra and in women who have an anteriorly retracted urethral meatus.[1,2] For straight catheterization needed only for a urine sample or to empty the bladder a single time, the length of the tube should be 6″ to 8″ for women and 16″ for men.[2] When inserting an indwelling catheter, longer tubing is desired to allow for more comfortable positioning of the catheter bag.

Preparation and Patient Positioning

A urinary catheterization kit contains, at minimum, the urinary catheter, sterile lubricant, and a sterilizing solution to clean the genitals before insertion. Sterile gloves and a 5 to 10 mL saline flush to inflate the balloon should also be obtained. Although urinary catheterization is typically performed as a sterile procedure, data comparing sterile technique against a clean technique in which the genitals are cleaned with water before insertion do not support increased risk of urinary tract infection in the clean technique.[3]

Female patients are placed in a supine position with the soles of the feet together while letting the knees fall to the sides. If body habitus or comorbidities limit this position, dorsal lithotomy positioning with stirrups can also be used. Male patients are placed supine with legs extended.

Procedural approach[4,5]
- Open the kit and arrange on a sterile field. The tip of the catheter should be coated in sterile lubricant.
- Female patients: using the nondominant hand spread the labia majora and minora apart until adequate visualization of the urethra is achieved.

Male patients: using the nondominant hand grasp the penis and pull gently upward at a 90° angle from the body to straighten the urethra. If foreskin is obscuring the urethra gentle downward traction is applied until the urethra is adequately visualized.
The nondominant hand will stay in place for the duration of the procedure.

- Clean the urethral opening with the cleansing solution contained in the kit.
- Bring the lubricated tip of the catheter to the urethral opening and advance. If resistance is met, retract slightly and attempt to advance again. Do not use excessive force to move past resistance. For male patients, if increased resistance occurs at the point of the bulbar urethra, the penis may be directed downward to the patient's feet to allow passage through the prostatic urethra.[1]
- For in-and-out catheterization, the catheter can be removed once urine return is noted and the sample collected. If placing an indwelling catheter in female patients, advance the catheter 2 to 3 cm past the point of urine return, then inflate the balloon. In male patients, the entire length of the catheter should be inserted before inflation of the balloon.
- After the balloon is inflated with 5 to 10 mL saline, gently pull on the catheter tubing until resistance is met to ensure the catheter is securely within the bladder.

Management and Outcomes

For indwelling urinary catheters, visible debris should be removed from the catheter daily, but use of antibiotic ointments or sterilizing soaps and washes on the tubing has not been shown to decrease risk of urinary tract infection.[3] Before removal of an indwelling catheter for urinary retention, a voiding trial may be attempted to predict the risk of success of discontinuation.

Challenges

Urethral stricture, benign prostatic hyperplasia, infection, and inflammation may all make insertion more challenging. Excessive force used to overcome resistance due to these and other causes may cause urethral trauma.[1] If resistance cannot be overcome by repositioning or upsizing French size consider referral to urology or emergency services if urgent bladder drainage is needed.

Deflation of the catheter balloon may result in cuffing or folding of the plastic, which may make removal difficult and painful. Passive deflation of the balloon may lessen cuffing. If resistance or significant pain is met after deflation of the balloon, consider adding 0.5 mL back into the balloon to smooth cuffing and make removal easier and less painful.[6] In the event of a balloon that will not deflate, referral to urology is warranted.

SUPRAPUBIC CATHETER REPLACEMENT
Introduction

An SPC is an alternative means of bladder drainage that is used when clean intermittent catheterization (CIC) or an indwelling urinary catheter may not be appropriate, including permanent or insurmountable urologic obstruction or stricture, neurogenic bladder, or individuals who may suffer from pressure injury from chronically sitting on catheter tubing. For individuals with these conditions SPC may offer improved quality of life due to ease of management compared with CIC or indwelling catheter.[7] An SPC is initially placed by a surgeon skilled in insertion, but after initial healing an SPC may be changed by the patient, by home health nurse, or in the outpatient setting.

Anatomy

The stoma for an SPC will be in the midline lower abdomen above the pubic symphysis. The tract runs through the abdominal wall and detrusor muscle of the bladder into the bladder lumen.[8]

Preprocedure Planning and Patient Positioning

The stoma should be inspected for any signs of infection or skin breakdown. All materials for SPC exchange should be gathered and readily available, including new SPC and catheter bag and 10-mL saline syringe. Lubricating gel can also be used if needed. Should skin breakdown around the stoma be noted, use of lubricating gel including lidocaine is not recommended due to increased risk for systemic absorption.[8] Some patients may prefer a dressing be placed over the area, but this is not required. The patient should be placed supine and the area of the SPC well visualized.

Procedural approach[1,8]
- Clean the area around the SPC with saline.
- Deflate the catheter balloon and grip the catheter at the site of insertion.
- Gently retract the tube while maintaining the grip on the tube from the site of insertion.
- Resistance during removal is thought to be caused by detrusor muscle stimulation and contraction. Should resistance be met gently rotate the tube or place 2 fingers at the stoma site and press down gently.
- Once the catheter is removed note the distance from the tip of the catheter to the insertion site.
- Grasp the new catheter the same distance as was noted from the removed SPC.
- Insert the new catheter into the cystostomy tract to the approximate length noted from the prior catheter.
- Inflate the catheter balloon with 3 to 5 mL saline. If significant resistance is met or felt by the patient the catheter may have to be withdrawn or advanced slightly. If no resistance is met, gently pull back on the catheter to feel the balloon anchor against the bladder wall, and then completely inflate.

Complications and Management

Exchange of an SPC in primary care settings should occur with well-established cystostomy tracts. Although most risk of adverse events associated with SPC occur with initial placement, rarely complications such as bowel perforation can occur during routine change. Other complications that may occur include inflation of the balloon within the urethra or within the bladder wall.[7] Estimation of the length of tube from the previous catheter can help reduce this risk by protecting against reinsertion at too shallow or too deep a position with the replacement. Another common complication of SPC change is balloon cuffing. When a catheter balloon is deflated, creases or folds may occur in the material due to prolonged distension of the material.[9] As the balloon is retracted against the bladder wall these folds can cuff around the tube creating increased resistance as well as pain and bleeding. Slow removal of the balloon can reduce cuffing and increase patient comfort.[8,9] Finally, if an SPC is removed but a new catheter is not able to be replaced in a timely manner, excessive force must not be used to replace it[8]; this may result in complication such as insertion outside of the stoma tract. In this case referral to urology or an emergency department where urology can be accessed is warranted because the stoma tract may have closed or become occluded.

EXCISION OF THROMBOSED EXTERNAL HEMORRHOIDS
Introduction

The prevalence of hemorrhoids in the general population is estimated to be 40% to 80%, although fewer than half of affected individuals become symptomatic.[10] A minority of patients with anal symptoms spontaneously report their symptoms to their primary care physician.[11] Many symptomatic hemorrhoids can be managed conservatively with topical agents such as anti-inflammatories or nitroglycerin, bulking agents such as dietary fiber, and reassurance. Relatively few internal hemorrhoids require surgical intervention, whereas many thrombosed external hemorrhoids require evacuation or excision for symptomatic relief.

Anatomy

In healthy individuals, arteriovenous vessels in the proximal anal canal form a vascular cushion, which helps maintain fecal continence. These vessels are termed hemorrhoids when they bleed or protrude and are analogous to a varicose vein. The dentate (or pectinate) line is located 3 to 4 cm proximal to the anal verge and represents the junction of the proximal and distal segments of the anal canal, which have different embryonic origins. Internal hemorrhoids protrude from rectal mucosa proximal to the dentate line, which lacks innervation by somatic nerves. Thus, internal hemorrhoids are painless, whereas external hemorrhoids, those that arise from below the dentate line, can be exquisitely painful.

The rectum is divided into 8 segments. The longitudinal vessels of the anal canal typically align with the right posterior, right anterior, and left lateral segments. These segments, accordingly, are the typical sites of hemorrhoidal disease (**Fig. 1**).

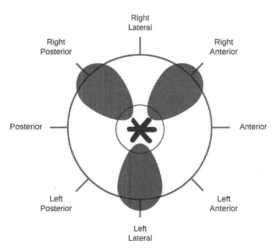

Fig. 1. The rectum is divided into 8 segments. Posterior corresponds to the superior gluteal cleft with the patient in the left lateral decubitus position. The right posterior, right anterior, and left lateral segments are the typical sites of hemorrhoidal disease. (*Courtesy of* Michael Firnhaber, PhD, Boulder, CO.)

Diagnosis

A thrombosed external hemorrhoid is easily recognized on physical examination as a firm, tender bluish purple nodule at the anal verge. Before surgical intervention, coexisting anal pathology, such as perianal abscess, should be excluded. Anoscopic evaluation may be performed after administration of local anesthesia if the area is highly tender.

Preprocedure Planning

The primary decision point when considering surgical removal of a thrombosed external hemorrhoid is time since onset of symptoms. Within the first 72 hours, the pain relief provided by a surgical procedure outweighs the discomfort of the procedure itself. Excision of thrombosed external hemorrhoids offers quicker resolution of symptoms, a lower risk of recurrence, and longer intervals of remission.[12] Without intervention, a thrombosed external hemorrhoid will resorb, fibrose, and ultimately resolve over 7 to 10 days.

Procedural approach
- The patient is positioned in the left lateral decubitus position with the right hip and knee flexed. An assistant may be necessary to retract the right buttock and allow adequate visualization of the anal field.
- The hemorrhoid and perianal skin are prepped with an antiseptic solution.
- The base of the hemorrhoid is infiltrated with 1 to 3 mL 2% lidocaine with epinephrine via a 25- or 27-gauge needle. The initial site of needle placement should be chosen to avoid the need for multiple needle punctures. The base of the hemorrhoid should blanch with anesthetic infiltration; a deeply placed needle may not provide adequate anesthesia.
- The entire external portion of the hemorrhoid, or the external surface of the hemorrhoid, is excised using a No. 15 blade and a fusiform incision. Most clinicians prefer a radially oriented incision, but a circumferential incision may be appropriate for lesions with a more circumferential orientation.
- Alternatively, a simple radial incision, without removal of overlying skin, may be performed. This approach may be appropriate for lesions presenting closer to the 72-h point, when the clot is better organized. The risk of reaccumulation is greater with this approach.
- Irrespective of the surgical approach, care must be taken to express and evacuate all clot contained within the hemorrhoid. Mosquito hemostats are helpful to explore and break through any remaining septa that may cover residual clot.
- Focused electrocautery may be used for hemostasis if direct pressure alone does not control bleeding.
- In most cases, the surgical site is left open to heal by secondary intention. Larger excisions may be closed with 4-0 or 5-0 absorbable subcutaneous sutures.
- The wound is then inspected for hemostasis, antibiotic ointment is applied, and a gauze pad is tucked between the buttocks for additional direct pressure.

Recovery/postprocedure care
- Sitz baths several times per day for 5 to 7 days postprocedure.
- Stool softeners, fiber supplement, and adequate fluid intake can help prevent hard stools and associated straining with defecation.
- Oral analgesics and topical anesthetics, such as 5% lidocaine jelly, are particularly helpful in the first few days.
- Routine follow-up in 4 to 6 weeks is appropriate.

- A long-term bowel regimen can decrease the risk of recurrent symptomatic hemorrhoidal disease.

CLINICS CARE POINTS

- Urinary catheterization can be safely performed in primary care settings to relieve urinary tract obstruction or to obtain urine samples.
- Careful attention should be paid to anatomy and prior history of urethral instrumentation or stricture to avoid traumatic catheterization.
- Larger French sizes may be used in cases of benign prostatic hyperplasia to facilitate insertion through the prostatic urethra.
- SPC replacement in primary care settings should only be performed with well-established cystostomy tracts.
- There are multiple different approaches to SPC replacement, but estimation of the depth of insertion based on prior SPC is a reliable and efficient method for replacement that can be performed by the patient or in primary care settings.
- The primary decision point when considering surgical removal of a thrombosed external hemorrhoid is time since onset of symptoms.
- Within the first 72 hours of symptom onset, excision of thrombosed external hemorrhoids offers quicker resolution of symptoms, a lower risk of recurrence, and longer intervals of remission.
- Simple radial incision and clot evacuation is associated with a greater risk of reaccumulation than if complete excision is performed.

DISCLOSURE

The authors have nothing to disclose.

REFERENCES

1. Bianchi A, Chesnut GT. Difficult foley catheterization. In: StatPearls [Internet]. Treasure Island (FL): StatPearls Publishing; 2020.
2. Beauchemin L, Newman DK, Le Danseur M, et al. Best practices for clean intermittent catheterization. Nursing 2018;48(9):49–54.
3. Moola S, Konno R. A systematic review of the management of short-term indwelling urethral catheters to prevent urinary tract infections. JBI Libr Syst Rev 2010;8(17):695–729.
4. Cancio LC, Sabanegh ES Jr, Thompson IM. Managing the Foley catheter. Am Fam Physician 1993;48(5):829–36.
5. Thomsen TW, Setnik GS. Videos in clinical medicine. Male urethral catheterization. N Engl J Med 2006;354(21):e22.
6. Patterson R, Little B, Tolan J, et al. How to manage a urinary catheter balloon that will not deflate. Int Urol Nephrol 2006;38(1):57–61.
7. Hunter KF, Bharmal A, Moore KN. Long-term bladder drainage: Suprapubic catheter versus other methods: a scoping review. Neurourol Urodyn 2013;32(7): 944–51.
8. Robinson J. Clinical skills: how to remove and change a suprapubic catheter. Br J Nurs 2005;14(1):30–5.

9. Robinson J. Suprapubic catheter removal: the cuffing effect of deflated catheter balloons. Br J Community Nurs 2003;8(5):205–8.
10. Riss S, Weiser FA, Schwameis K, et al. The prevalence of hemorrhoids in adults. Int J Colorectal Dis 2012;27(2):215–20.
11. Tournu G, Abramowitz L, Couffignal C, et al. Prevalence of anal symptoms in general practice: a prospective study. Bmc Fam Pract 2017;18(1):78.
12. Greenspon J, Williams SB, Young HA, et al. Thrombosed external hemorrhoids: outcome after conservative or surgical management. Dis Colon Rectum 2004; 47(9):1493–8.

ADDITIONAL REFERENCES

Davis BR, Lee-Kong SA, Migaly J, et al. The American Society of Colon and Rectal Surgeons Clinical Practice Guidelines for the Management of Hemorrhoids. Dis Colon Rectum 2018;61(3):284–92.

Jongen J, Bach S, Stübinger SH, et al. Excision of Thrombosed External Hemorrhoid Under Local Anesthesia. Dis Colon Rectum 2003;46(9):1226–31.

Solomon CG, Jacobs D. Hemorrhoids. N Engl J Med 2014;371(10):944–51.

Wald A, Bharucha AE, Cosman BC, et al. ACG Clinical Guideline: Management of Benign Anorectal Disorders. Am J Gastroenterol 2014;109(8):1141–57.

Laboratory and Diagnostic Light Office Procedures

Annie Rutter, MD, MS[a],*, Madeline Haas, MD[b]

KEYWORDS

- Wood's lamp • Microscope • Office microscopy • Vaginitis/vaginal discharge
- Potassium hydroxide (KOH) preparation • Fluorescein • Wet prep/wet mount
- Urine sediment

KEY POINTS

- Office-based diagnostic tests using a microscope or ultraviolet diagnostic light can aid in the diagnosis of several common ambulatory care concerns including vaginal discharge and skin rash.
- Microscopy using the Amsel criteria is the test of choice for diagnosis of bacterial vaginosis.
- Urine sediment examination using centrifuge in combination with office microscopy can evaluate acute and chronic kidney disease and is often superior to automated urinalysis.
- Skin evaluation with Wood's lamp demonstrating presence or absence of fluorescence, its color, and distribution aids in the diagnosis of tinea, erythrasma, and pigmentation disorders.
- In conjunction with other elements of an ophthalmologic assessment, fluorescein and a Wood's lamp can be used to diagnose corneal abrasion.

INTRODUCTION

Office-based and bedside diagnostic procedures can be a helpful tool when assessing patients in the ambulatory setting. The diagnostic tests discussed here are useful because they are easy to perform in a short period of time and aid in diagnostic certainty. Additionally, much of the equipment is a one-time or infrequent investment with minimal ancillary resources making it cost-effective. A microscope and/or a diagnostic UV light (or Wood's lamp) can be used to assess a multitude of patient presentations including, but not limited to,

[a] Department of Family & Community Medicine, Albany Medical College, 43 New Scotland Avenue, Albany, NY 12208, USA; [b] Department of Family & Community Medicine, Albany Medical College, 391 Myrtle Avenue, Suite 4B, Albany, NY 12208, USA
* Corresponding author.
E-mail address: Ruttera@amc.edu

Prim Care Clin Office Pract 48 (2021) 685–705
https://doi.org/10.1016/j.pop.2021.07.007
0095-4543/21/© 2021 Elsevier Inc. All rights reserved.

- Vaginitis (vaginal discharge, odor, itching, or pain)
- Skin rashes/lesions
- Eye pain
- Urinary symptoms
- Clinical findings suggestive of acute kidney injury (AKI) or chronic kidney disease (CKD).

MICROSCOPY

Many primary care offices include an office-based laboratory with microscopy, which operates under a Clinical Laboratory Improvement Amendments of 1988 (CLIA) certificate. Provider-performed microscopy allows for health care providers to perform moderate-complexity tests as part of the patient examination, prioritizing specimens that deteriorate quickly or cannot be easily transported. Additionally, office-based microscopy is inexpensive and offers point-of-care diagnosis. Microscopy is commonly used for wet mount and potassium hydroxide (KOH) preparations, fern tests, urine sediment, semen analysis, and other tests. Bright-field microscopy illuminates the specimen with bright white light, retaining the specimen's natural colors, and can magnify up to 40x. Specialized objectives allow for phase-contrast microscopy, which illustrates cellular elements not seen with standard bright-light microscopy. CLIA-certified laboratories must have a director and competency standards for providers.[1]

Vaginal Discharge

Patients with symptoms of vaginitis, including vaginal discharge, odor, itching, pain, or redness,[2] should undergo examination that includes microscopy, as a medical history alone has been found to be insufficient for diagnosis.[3,4] All women with a complaint of vaginal discharge should be tested for trichomoniasis.[4] Office-based microscopy offers advantages of point-of-care diagnosis and cost-effectiveness.[2-4]

Asymptomatic women should not be screened or treated for vaginitis, including those with pathogens noted on Pap smear.[3] There is a high prevalence of naturally occurring bacterial and *Candida* species in normal vaginal flora of asymptomatic women (20% and 12%–13%, respectively),[2,3] in contrast to a very low prevalence of trichomoniasis (no cases in one study of 100 patients).[2] Trichomoniasis screening may be considered in high-prevalence settings such as sexually transmitted infection (STI) clinics and correctional facilities.[4]

Vaginal flora is estrogen-dependent and, in the reproductive years, includes lactobacilli as well as numerous species including *Gardnerella vaginalis*, *Escherichia coli*, group B *streptococci*, genital *Mycoplasma* species, and *Candida albicans*, among others.[3,5] Estrogen increases glycogen content in vaginal epithelial cells, leading to lactobacillus colonization, which produce lactic acid that lowers the vaginal pH to less than 4.5. This acidic environment protects against bacterial overgrowth and other pathogens.[3,5,6]

Prepubertal and postmenopausal females lack estrogen to support the vaginal bacterial ecosystem. In these women, microscopy shows few epithelial cells, lactobacilli, or background bacteria, and pH is greater than 4.5. As a result, bacterial vaginosis and *Candida* infections are less common in these populations.[3]

Bacterial vaginosis is caused by an overgrowth of numerous anaerobic bacteria (including *Gardnerella vaginalis*, *Mycoplasma*, *Bacteroides*, and many others) and a lack of lactobacilli.[3-5] Estimates of the prevalence of bacterial vaginosis, vaginal candidiasis, and trichomoniasis among symptomatic patients range from 22% to 50%, 17% to 39%, and 4% to 35%, respectively.[3] Up to 49% of women report at least one lifetime episode of vaginal candidiasis.[3]

Trichomoniasis is the most common nonviral STI in the United States, with over 3 million infections annually.[3,4] According to the Centers for Disease Control and Prevention, "health disparities persist in the epidemiology of trichomoniasis: Thirteen percent of Black women are affected compared with 1.8% of non-Hispanic White women." Trichomoniasis also has high prevalence among patients seen in STI clinics and people who are incarcerated.[4]

Diagnosis
Bacterial vaginosis. Microscopy using the Amsel criteria is the test of choice for diagnosis of bacterial vaginosis, with a sensitivity of up to 92% to 98% compared with the reference standard (Gram stain with Nugent scoring)[2,3] and a specificity of 77%.[3] Polymerase chain reaction and DNA probe are of limited utility as numerous organisms can cause bacterial vaginosis.[3]

Bacterial vaginosis is diagnosed with three of four Amsel criteria[3,7]:

1. Homogeneous, thin, watery discharge that smoothly coats the vaginal walls
2. Vaginal epithelial cells with over 20% "clue cells" on a saline-solution slide
3. Vaginal fluid pH above 4.5
4. Positive KOH amine or "whiff test"

When microscopy is not available, the original Amsel criteria can be fulfilled by patient complaint of vaginal discharge, findings of elevated pH, and positive "whiff test" result,[3] with sensitivity of 80% and specificity of 91% in one study of patients who meet two of three criteria.[8]

Candidiasis. Candidiasis may be diagnosed either by (1) microscopy or Gram stain or (2) a culture or commercial test positive for *Candida* species.[3,4] Wet mount with KOH preparation reveals spores, budding yeast, pseudohyphae, or hyphae, with a sensitivity of 50% to 60% and a specificity of 89% in one study.[8] Yeast is associated with a pH of less than 4.5.

Trichomoniasis. Trichomonads may be seen on vaginal wet preparation, although that is not the test of choice.[3] Vaginal wet mount has limited sensitivity (50%–75%),[2–4,8] which is lower in specimens from men,[4] and a specificity of up to 99%.[8] Trichomonads appear as flagellated, motile organisms.[9] Nucleic acid amplification (NAAT) is the preferred test for diagnosis of trichomonas infection, over commercial tests or culture, with an estimated sensitivity and specificity of 95% to 100%, and can be obtained on vaginal, urine, or semen samples.[3]

Procedure
Materials
- Speculum
- Sterile lubrication jelly
- Sterile cotton-tipped 8-inch swab
- Additional swabs as needed for *Trichomonas vaginalis* NAAT or *Candida* culture
- Collection dish or test tube
- Narrow range pH paper
- 1 mL sterile saline
- 1 mL KOH 10%
- 1 slide

- 2 slide covers
- Microscope

Examination. Begin by examining the patient's vulva in the lithotomy position.[3,6,9] Bacterial vaginosis does not affect the vulva, whereas *Candida* and trichomoniasis may lead to vulvar erythema, edema, excoriations, and fissures.[3,6]

Then, insert a lubricated speculum to the cervix.[6,9] Inspect the cervix, fornices, and vaginal walls. A thick white vaginal discharge is characteristic of *Candida*, whereas a yellow-green bubbly discharge suggests trichomoniasis.[3]

Obtaining samples. Gently apply the cotton-tipped swab directly to the vaginal fornices and side walls to collect a sample.[3] To assess vaginal pH, apply the swab to pH paper (**Fig. 1**).[6] The examiner may also apply pH paper directly to nondilute discharge obtained from the vaginal side wall or from the speculum after removal.[9] Cervical mucus, blood, semen, lubricants, and other substances may all falsely elevate the pH.[3]

Place the cotton-tipped swab into a labeled collection dish or test tube containing 0.5-1 mL of normal saline.[6,9] Collect additional swabs as needed for NAAT or culture and remove the speculum.[6] Sensitivity is highest with immediate examination under a microscope,[4] within 10 minutes.[4,6]

Preparing samples. In the laboratory space, mix the swab in approximately 1 mL of saline solution, then remove the swab and press it gently onto a slide. Apply a coverslip and examine immediately.

To prepare the KOH sample, first press the saline swab onto the slide as mentioned previously and then add one drop of 10% KOH solution. A "whiff test" is then performed by smelling the solution before adding a coverslip.[6] Allow the KOH sample to air dry before examination under the microscopy. The 10% KOH serves to disrupt cells that might otherwise obscure *Candida* findings.[4]

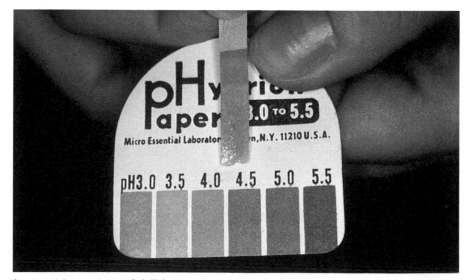

Fig. 1. pH Paper. *From* Abdallah, M. Vulvovaginitis and Cervicitis. In: *Mandell, Douglas, and Bennett's Principles and Practice of Infectious Diseases.* 9th ed. Elsevier; 2020; with permission.

One may examine the wet prep and KOH samples side by side on the same slide, with the wet prep examined first. Examine at least five fields first under low (10X) and then under high (40X) magnification.[9]

Interpreting findings. An elevated pH (greater than 4.5) is suggestive of bacterial vaginosis or trichomoniasis.[4]

A positive "whiff test" (an amine or fishy odor) suggests bacterial vaginosis.[7,9]

Examination of saline slide may reveal the following findings:

- Normal vaginal discharge is characterized by vaginal epithelial cells and lactobacilli (**Fig. 2**).[6]
- Lactobacilli, which appear as bacillary rods, may be absent or diminished in bacterial vaginosis.[9]
- Leukocytes at a concentration of more than 5 to 10 cells per high power field suggest cervicitis or other inflammatory process[4,9] and are less prevalent in bacterial vaginosis alone.[6]
- "Clue cells" are vaginal squamous epithelial cells with adherent coccobacilli, which often obscure the cell borders and nuclei (**Fig. 3**).[3,4,6,7,9]
- Trichomonads are anaerobic protozoans with motile flagella, about the same size as epithelial cells.[5,9] A warmer, more recently obtained sample is more likely to show motile organisms (**Fig. 4**).[6]

Examination of the 10% KOH slide:

- Budding yeast, spores, pseudohyphae, or hyphae (**Fig. 5**).

Discussion

Microscopy with application of Amsel criteria is the gold standard for diagnosis of bacterial vaginosis. If Amsel criteria are not met, no further testing or treatment is recommended.

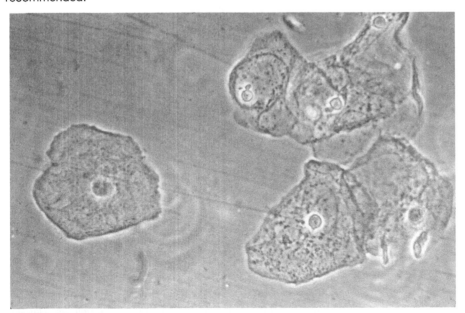

Fig. 2. Normal vaginal epithelial cells. *From* Abdallah, M. Vulvovaginitis and Cervicitis. In: *Mandell, Douglas, and Bennett's Principles and Practice of Infectious Diseases.* 9th ed. Elsevier; 2020; with permission.

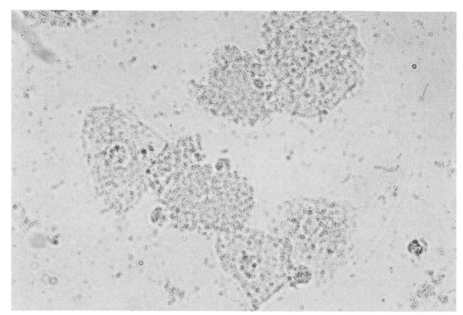

Fig. 3. Clue cells. *From* Abdallah, M. Vulvovaginitis and Cervicitis. In: *Mandell, Douglas, and Bennett's Principles and Practice of Infectious Diseases.* 9th ed. Elsevier; 2020; with permission.

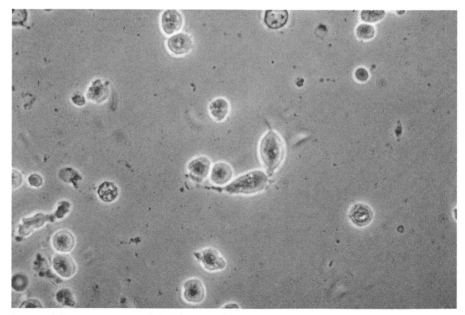

Fig. 4. Trichomonas. *From* Abdallah, M. Vulvovaginitis and Cervicitis. In: *Mandell, Douglas, and Bennett's Principles and Practice of Infectious Diseases.* 9th ed. Elsevier; 2020; with permission.

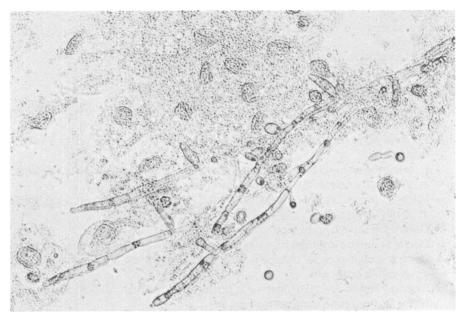

Fig. 5. Vulvovaginal candidiasis. *From* Abdallah, M. Vulvovaginitis and Cervicitis. In: *Mandell, Douglas, and Bennett's Principles and Practice of Infectious Diseases.* 9th ed. Elsevier; 2020; with permission.

Microscopy has limited sensitivity for *Candida* and trichomonas. If organisms are not seen under microscopy, additional testing with *Candida* culture or NAAT for trichomonas is appropriate.[2,4] *Candida* culture with speciation is also recommended for recurrent or resistant *Candida* infections.

Urine sediment

Microscopic examination of urine sediment is a useful tool in diagnosing the etiology of AKI as well as CKD. No finding is pathognomonic but must be combined with clinical history.[10] Urine sediment offers inexpensive, point-of-care testing; however, limitations include lack of provider knowledge and experience with the examination, which requires a centrifuge and must be performed in a CLIA-certified laboratory.[11,12]

Interobserver reliability among nephrologists may be as low as 59% to 69%.[13]

Diagnosis

Manual urine sediment is superior to automated urinalysis in diagnosis of acute tubular necrosis, glomerulonephritis, vasculitis, and crystalline kidney diseases.[10,12] Phase contrast microscopy is superior to bright field microscopy and is especially useful for identifying abnormal cells and casts,[14] while polarized light is required for viewing crystals.[15]

Procedure
Materials
- Sterile urine cup and wipes for the patient to obtain clean-catch urine
- Urine dipstick (pH and specific gravity)

- Test tube
- Microscope
- Centrifuge
- Suction pipette
- Glass slide and cover slip

Obtaining and Preparing Samples[10]

- Collect urine from a clean-catch spontaneous void; for patients with indwelling urinary catheters, urine should be drawn from the catheter tubing.
- Examine urine as quickly as possible, within 1 to 2 hours, or up to 8 hours if refrigerated.
- Examine the whole urine for color and clarity (vs turbidity) and use a urine dipstick or automatic analysis to measure pH and osmolality.
- Place 10 mL of urine into a test tube and centrifuge for at least 5 minutes at 1500 rpm or higher.
- Decant the urine by pouring or suctioning off 9.5 mL.
- Gently shake the test tube to resuspend the remaining 0.5 mL of urine sediment.
- Using a suction pipette, place one drop of urine sediment onto a glass slide and cover with a cover slip.
- Examine first at low (10x) then high power (40x), at least 10 fields total, using bright field or phase contrast microscopy.

Interpreting Findings. A urine dipstick to measure pH and specific gravity is required to contextualize microscopy findings: pH greater than 7 and specific gravity less than 1.010 may lead to lysis of erythrocytes and leukocytes and impairs cast formation, while specific gravity over 1.030 can reduce the sensitivity of urine dipstick for hemoglobin and leukocyte esterase.[15]

Cells A variety of cells can be visualized during specimen interpretation and can be a normal finding or suggestive of pathology (**Table 1**).

Noncell findings: lipids and crystals (**Table 2**) Cholesterol particles appear as round drops, oval fat bodies, fatty casts, or cholesterol crystals. Presence of lipids, especially when associated with proteinuria, suggests glomerular disease.[15]

Crystals must be viewed under polarized light with a known urine pH, as pH affects crystal precipitation. Examination for crystals is useful in assessing nephrolithiasis as well as suspected drug nephrotoxicity. Many types of crystals exist, including uric acid, calcium oxalate, calcium phosphate, cholesterol, drugs, and others. Persistent uric acid or calcium oxalate crystals can suggest increased urinary excretion of these elements, which can lead to stone formation. Uric acid crystals are nonspecific but can be seen in ethylene glycol intoxication. Phosphate crystals may be seen in certain types of urinary tract infections.[15]

Casts Casts form in the distal renal tubules and collecting ducts and may be formed by any of the elements noted previously. Hyaline casts are colorless, best seen with phase contrast microscopy, and can be a normal finding. Granular and hyaline-granular casts are pathologic and may be seen in glomerulonephritis, acute interstitial nephritis, and acute tubular necrosis. Waxy casts are nonspecific findings in AKI and CKD. Hemoglobin casts appear brown and granular; myoglobin casts have a similar appearance and are seen in rhabdomyolysis[15] (**Fig. 8**).

Discussion

Urine sediment is particularly useful in the following clinical scenarios:

Table 1
Cells found in urine sediment, appearance, and suggested disease origin

Finding	Appearance	Disease Origin
Erythrocytes and casts (**Fig. 6**)	Diameter ~6 μm; dysmorphic cells have irregular membranes	Dysmorphic and casts—glomerulus Isomorphic—urinary tract
Neutrophils (**Fig. 7**)	Diameter ~10 μm; granular cytoplasm, lobulated nucleus	Infection, acute interstitial nephritis, chronic interstitial nephritis, proliferative glomerulonephritis, external genitalia
Eosinophils	Special stain required	Acute allergic interstitial nephritis, infection, systemic inflammatory disease
Lymphocytes	Special stain required	Transplant rejection, chyluria
Macrophages	Mononucleated or multinucleated cells varying in size (13–95 μm diameter); may form oval fat bodies with lipids	Nonspecific
Renal tubular epithelial cells and casts	Variable size (diameter 9–25 μm) and shape (roundish or rectangular), central or peripheral large nucleus; may form casts	Acute tubular necrosis, acute interstitial nephritis, acute cellular rejection, and glomerular diseases
Transitional epithelial cells	Deep cells diameter ~18 μm, superficial diameter ~25 μm	Obstructive process (postrenal AKI), cystitis
Squamous epithelial cells	Diameter ~50 μm	Contamination with genital secretions

Data from Johnson RJ, Feehally J, Floege Jr. Comprehensive clinical nephrology. 6th ed. Elsevier; 2019.

Table 2
Noncell urinary sediment findings, appearance, and suggested disease origin

Finding	Appearance	Disease Origin
Lipids	Round, translucent, yellow drops of varying size, single or in clusters; may form oval fat bodies, fatty casts, or crystals. Polarized light reveals Maltese cross shape and nonbirefringent crystals.	Glomerular disease and nephrotic syndrome
Crystals	Precipitation varies with pH. Polarized light required: appearance varies depending on type.	Stone formation, drug toxicity
Casts	Cylindrical; appearance varies depending on content	Distal renal tubules and collecting ducts in a variety of conditions

Data from Johnson RJ, Feehally J, Floege Jr. Comprehensive clinical nephrology. 6th ed. Elsevier; 2019.

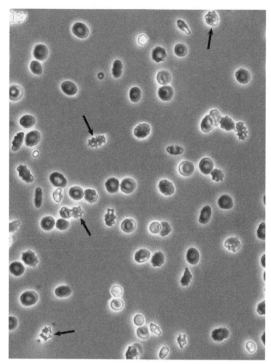

Fig. 6. Urine erythrocytes. The *arrows* indicate the so-called crenated erythrocytes, which are a finding in nonglomerular hematuria.[15] (image by phase contrast microscopy; original magnification ×400). *From* Johnson RJ, Feehally J, Floege Jr. Comprehensive clinical nephrology. 6th ed. Elsevier; 2019; with permission.

- Distinguishing acute tubular necrosis from prerenal AKI. Greater prevalence of renal tubular epithelial cells and their casts is associated with greater likelihood of acute tubular necrosis.[12,15]
- A bland urine sediment (without cellular components) and hyaline casts suggests prerenal AKI.[12]
- Dysmorphic erythrocytes and their casts suggest glomerular injury, which may lead to referral to a nephrologist rather than a urologist.[12]
- In the absence of a positive urine culture, leukocytes and their casts may suggest tubulointerstitial disease.[12]
- Cholesterol particles, especially when associated with proteinuria, suggests nephrotic syndrome or glomerular disease.[12,15]

Examination of urine sediment can be useful when attempting to determine the underlying cause of AKI or CKD (**Table 3**).

Skin scraping

Visualization of skin samples under microscopy can aid in the diagnosis of several skin conditions. Preparation of skin scales with KOH on a slide for microscopic evaluation can aid in the diagnosis of tinea infections, or when ruling out dermatophyte infections for lesions that may have a similar clinical appearance (such as nummular eczema).[16] It can also be used to diagnose yeast infections, such as *Candida*. When the

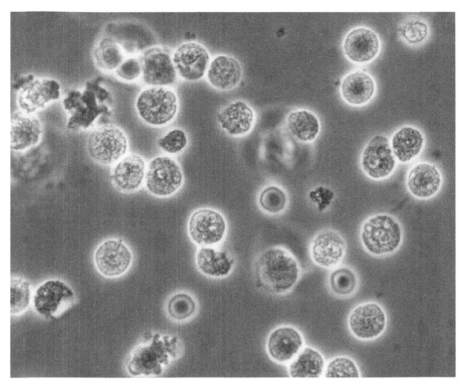

Fig. 7. Urine neutrophils (image by phase contrast microscopy; original magnification ×400). *From* Johnson RJ, Feehally J, Floege Jr. Comprehensive clinical nephrology. 6th ed. Elsevier; 2019; with permission.

differential diagnosis includes scabies, the use of microscopy with oil immersion can allow for the direct visualization of mites, ova, or scybala (fecal matter).[17]

Skin mycosis is a common problem globally, with a prevalence of 20% to 25%.[18] Scabies has an incidence of 300 million cases annually and carries with it a risk of severe outbreaks in places such as nursing homes and hospitals.[19]

Diagnosis
Direct visualization of branching hyphae in keratinized material is the gold standard for diagnosis of dermatophyte infections of the skin.[20] Using a KOH preparation with microscopy to do this can be carried out in many office settings. In one study of tinea pedis, a KOH preparation had a sensitivity of 73.3% and specificity of 42.5%, when using clinical assessment as the gold standard.[21] Direct visualization of mites or eggs with oil immersion microscopy is the gold standard for diagnosis of scabies.[22] Sensitivity of this examination is approximately 50%.[22,23]

Procedure
Materials
- Microscope
- #10 or #15 scalpel blade
- Glass slide
- KOH (5%-20% solution)[20]
- Mineral oil

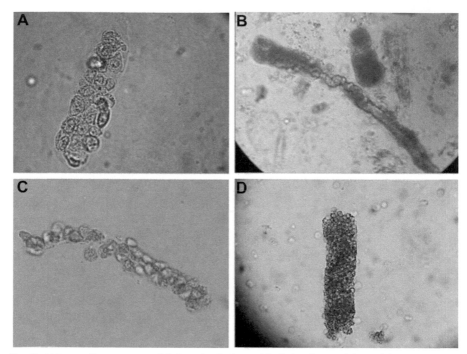

Fig. 8. Urine sediment: casts. (*A*) Renal tubular epithelial cell cast. (*B*) Muddy brown granular cast. (*C*) White blood cell cast. (*D*) Red blood cell cast. *From* Perazella MA. The urine sediment as a biomarker of kidney disease. Am J Kidney Dis. 2015 Nov;66(5):748 to 55; with permission.

- Cover slip
- Heat source

Examination. Position the patient so that you can easily visualize the area of concern. Place the scalpel perpendicular to the skin surface and draw the blade against the scale.[20] Place the slide underneath the blade so all scale falls onto the slide. It is best to obtain the sample from the leading edge of the lesion.[20,24]

- If assessing for dermatophytes: Place one drop of KOH preparation onto the sample and lay the cover slip on top. Heat the bottom of the slide slightly to warm the sample. Visualize under microscope.
- If assessing for scabies: Place a small amount (one drop) of mineral oil on skin area of concern before scraping. Scrape using the same technique as mentioned previously onto the slide. Place cover slip and visualize under the microscope.[17]

Interpreting findings. Microscopic visualization of mites, ova, or scybala confirms the diagnosis of scabies (**Fig. 9**). Budding cells and pseudohyphae are commonly described as "spaghetti and meatballs" and are indicative of fungal infection (**Fig. 10**), including *Candida*.[24]

Discussion
Direct visualization of scabies mites (or ova or scybala) or hyphae is sufficient to diagnose each infection. When coupled with clinical suspicion, appropriate treatment can

Table 3
Common renal injuries and the associated urine sediment findings

Etiology of Renal Injury	Characteristics	Absent or Minimal	Urine Dipstick
Prerenal acute kidney injury	Hyaline casts	Cellular elements	
Acute tubular necrosis	Renal tubular epithelial cells and casts, granular casts, muddy brown casts		Protein variable
Nephrotic syndrome	Cholesterol particles and casts, renal tubular epithelial cells, hyaline and granular casts	Erythrocytes or leukocytes	Protein
Nephritic syndrome	Erythrocytes and leukocytes and casts, hemoglobin casts		Protein, blood
Acute interstitial nephritis	Leukocytes, renal tubular epithelial cells, erythrocytes, and casts	Negative urine culture	Leukocyte esterase, blood
Crystal nephropathy	Crystals, renal tubular epithelial cells, erythrocytes, leukocytes		Blood variable, leukocyte esterase variable
Rhabdomyolysis	Myoglobin casts		
Urinary tract infection	Organisms and leukocytes and casts, transitional epithelial cells, struvite crystals		Leukocyte esterase, nitrites, blood variable

Data from Refs 10 and 15.

be rendered immediately without waiting for further confirmatory testing, such as fungal culture.

DIAGNOSTIC UV LIGHT (WOOD'S LAMP)

Long-wave UV light can be used to assist in the diagnosis of multiple skin and hair conditions including erythrasma, tinea, and vitiligo.[25] It can also be used in the assessment of corneal abrasions and lesions when used in conjunction with fluorescein application.[24] An uncommon use is to assess for porphyria cutanea tarda by viewing a urine sample under UV light, which will fluoresce as a bright pink-orange color.[25] When used for these diagnostic purposes, the UV light is at a peak wavelength of 365 nm, and the area of concern is visualized through a filtered glass, typically with magnification. It is the characteristic fluorescence observed (or not observed) that aids the examiner in determining a likely diagnosis. While outside of the scope of this discussion, UV light can also be used as part of the assessment of potential sexual assault and may detect ejaculate or highlight areas on the body from which to collect samples for further evaluation.[25]

Corneal assessment

When patients present with eye complaints, it is important to determine if treatment in a primary care setting is appropriate or if immediate referral to an ophthalmologist for more intensive testing and treatment is necessary. If there is a history of penetrating

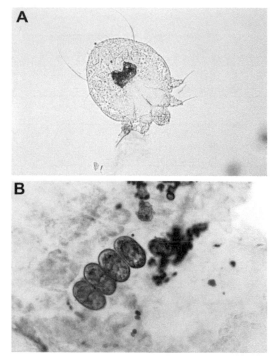

Fig. 9. Scabies. (*A*) Mites. (*B*) Ova and scybala. *From* Kliegman R, Stanton B, St. Geme JW, III, Schor NF, Behrman RE, Nelson WE. Nelson textbook of pediatrics. 21st ed. Elsevier; 2020; with permission.

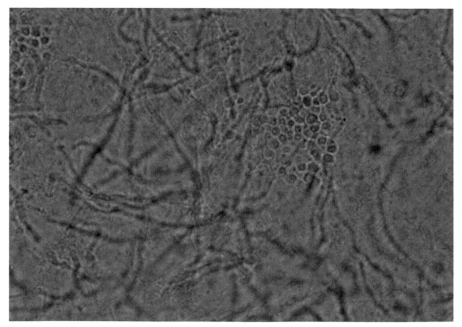

Fig. 10. KOH prep of skin scraping showing the "spaghetti and meatball" pattern of tinea versicolor. *From* Dinulos JGH. Habif's clinical dermatology: a color guide to diagnosis and therapy. 7th edition. Elsevier; 2019, with permission.

eye trauma or vision loss or, on initial examination, evidence of hyphema or pupillary irregularity (fixed, dilated, or irregular), urgent referral is warranted.[26,27] In the absence of these concerns, and with patient-reported symptoms of eye redness, tearing, sensitivity to light, or foreign body sensation, an evaluation in the primary care setting with Wood's lamp and fluorescein is an appropriate first step. Corneal abrasion, with or without presence of a foreign body, can be diagnosed with this technique.

Corneal abrasions or foreign bodies are not uncommon ocular injuries. With an annual incidence in the United States of approximately 0.2% to 0.3%, care is sought by these patients in both the emergency room and ambulatory setting.[28] Risk factors for corneal abrasion specifically include history of trauma, contact lens use, male gender, age between 20 and 34 years, construction or manufacturing job, and lack of eye protection.[27]

Diagnosis
The sensitivity of Wood's lamp evaluation is approximately 56% when used to detect corneal abrasions.[29] The sensitivity of the evaluation in the diagnosis of corneal ulcers or corneal foreign bodies is 50% and 44%, respectively. These diagnoses require different treatments and follow-up, and there is concern for long-term consequences if left undiagnosed. While a slit lamp evaluation is ideal, the use of a Wood's lamp is acceptable in resource-limited settings, and when the history is consistent with simple corneal abrasion and correlates with positive findings on fluorescein assessment.[29]

Procedure
Materials
- Topical ophthalmic anesthetic drops (eg, proparacaine or tetracaine)
- Wood's lamp
- Fluorescein-impregnated strip
  - Alternative: topical anesthetic drops premixed with fluorescein dye.[27]

Examination. It is important to perform the other elements of the ophthalmologic assessment before evaluation with fluorescein.[27] Visual acuity, fundoscopy, pupillary assessment, and inspection of conjunctival sacs are part of a comprehensive eye examination but may also reveal findings requiring more urgent evaluation by an ophthalmologist. If a Wood's lamp is not immediately available, a cobalt-blue filter (found on many ophthalmoscopes) can be used for this examination.[24,26]

- Place the patient in a supine position near an outlet where the UV light can be used.
- Instill topical anesthetic.
- Moisten the dry fluorescein strip by touching this strip to the tear pool anterior to bulbar conjunctiva.
- Have the patient blink several times to distribute the dye.
- Darken the room and examine the eye under UV light.[24,26]

Interpreting findings. Denuded or dead corneal epithelium will be green under either cobalt-blue light or Wood's lamp[24] (**Fig. 11**). In some cases, determining the underlying cause of the disruption of corneal epithelium can be suggested by the shape of the defect (**Table 4**).

Discussion
Corneal assessment with Wood's lamp is an important tool in the primary care ambulatory toolkit; however, it must be used in the proper clinical setting and in conjunction with other elements of a complete ophthalmologic assessment. Corneal abrasions

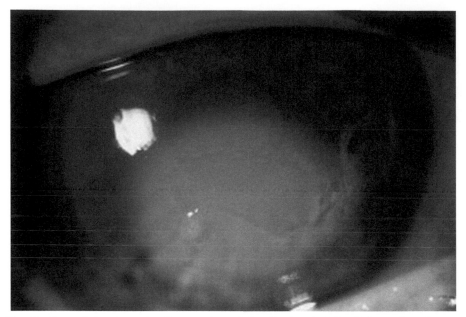

Fig. 11. Corneal abrasion using fluorescein and visualized under Wood's lamp. *From* Buttar-avoli PM, Leffler SM. Minor emergencies. 3rd ed. Elsevier; 2012; with permission.

can be accompanied by true foreign bodies, not just a foreign body sensation, and therefore, removal and irrigation needs to be arranged to prevent further injury, which may include scarring and vision loss.[26] The differential diagnosis of eye irritation can be broad, and if history or physical examination findings suggest the issue is more chronic, proper follow-up and treatment of the underlying cause is needed.

Skin lesions or rashes

Diagnostic UV light can aid in the diagnosis of a multitude of skin conditions including those characterized by abnormal pigmentation, hair loss, blisters, or dermatitis (especially when located in body folds).[25,30,31] In addition to assistance with diagnosis, a UV light can also assess for evenness of application of chemical peels on the skin,

Table 4
Causes of denuded cornea suggested by shape of lesion

Diagnosis	Finding
Traumatic corneal abrasion	Linear/geographic
Herpes Simplex keratitis	Dendritic, can also be geographic if large
Neurotropic (diabetic neuropathy, abuse of topical anesthetics, chronic contact lens wearer)	Geographic with rolled edges
Contact lens involvement	Punctate lesions surrounding round central defect.

Data from Refs 26 and 27.

Table 5
Skin diagnoses and corresponding findings under Wood's lamp

Diagnosis	Finding Under Wood's Lamp
Infections	
Fungal infections	
Tinea capitis	Black dot pattern when magnified
Trichophyton tonsurans	Does not fluoresce
Microsporum audouinii or *M. canis*	Yellow green (hair shaft, not skin)
Tinea versicolor	Golden yellow
Trichophyton	White-green
Erythrasma (*Corynebacterium minutissimum*)	Coral red
Pseudomonas	Aqua-green or white green
Pigmentation disorders	
Vitiligo	Hypopigmentation is accentuated
Tuberous sclerosis	Hypopigmentation of ash leaf spots is accentuated
Congenital dermal melanocytosis	No accentuation

Data from Refs 25 and 30.

specifically those containing salicylic acid.[25] The gold standard for many skin conditions is biopsy or, in the case of dermatophyte infections, visualization of hyphae.[20] However, bedside evaluation with Wood's lamp can provide quick and helpful diagnostic information.

Skin rashes and conditions are one of the top acute care diagnoses assessed in the ambulatory care setting.[32] Fungal infections of the nails and skin are common globally, with a prevalence of 20% to 25% of the world's population.[18] The clinician's ability to differentiate diseases such as erythrasma from dermatophyte infections may help promote earlier intervention and treatment. Pigmentation disorders have varied prevalence; vitiligo has a worldwide prevalence of 0.4% to 2%.[33] Congenital dermal melanocytosis varies by ethnicity with a prevalence of over 80% in Asian populations, 95% in Black populations, and nearly 10% in White populations.[34]

Diagnosis
As noted previously, findings on Wood's lamp assessment are not the gold standard for diagnosis of most skin conditions. Additionally, false positive (due to lint, soaps,

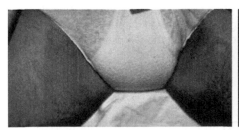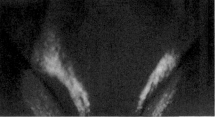

Fig. 12. Erythrasma: with and without Wood's lamp. *From* Fowler GC. Pfenninger & Fowler's procedures for primary care. 4th ed. Elsevier; 2020, with permission.

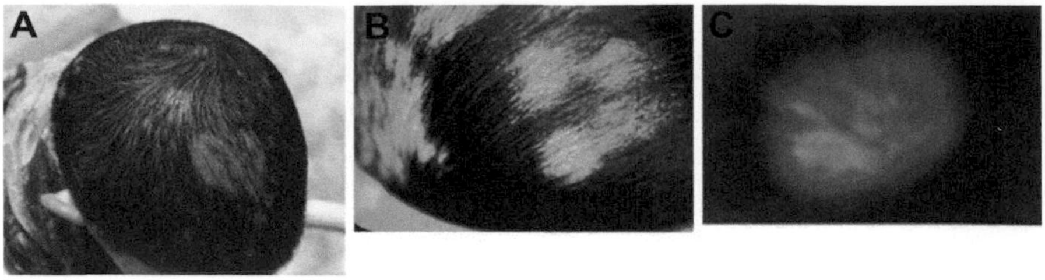

Fig. 13. Tinea capitis. *From* Fowler GC. Pfenninger & Fowler's procedures for primary care. 4th ed. Elsevier; 2020, with permission.

lotions, or other chemicals) and false negative results can occur.[25] The presence of fluorescence as well as its color and distribution aid in diagnosis.

Procedure
Materials

- Wood's lamp

Examination. Position the patient near an outlet so that the lamp can be plugged in and easily operated and repositioned to examine all areas of skin under investigation. Turn on the lamp and allow to "warm up" for a few minutes. Darken the room. Place the Wood's lamp 10 to 30 cm (approximately 8 inches) over the area of skin to be examined and observe the findings through the glass of the Wood's lamp.[25,31] Pay specific attention to the fluorescence observed including color and distribution.

It is important *not* to wash the skin before examination, ideally for the 24 hours preceding, to decrease the possibility of a false negative result.

Interpreting findings. Examiners should note the presence (or absence) of fluorescence and its color. In pigmentation disorders, the Wood's lamp can help accentuate truly amelanotic skin (**Table 5**; **Fig. 12** and **Fig. 13**).

Discussion
Wood's lamp assessment of skin rashes or lesions can be used in conjunction with clinical history to aid in the diagnosis of several skin conditions. Additionally, it can also assist in determining which areas of the skin to sample for further laboratory investigation.[31] While the test itself is not difficult to perform and does not require extensive amounts of equipment, proper interpretation can take time, training, and expertise.[31]

SUMMARY

Office-based testing using microscopy or diagnostic UV light (such as Wood's lamp) can be helpful in providing immediate diagnoses for common presenting concerns in the ambulatory care setting. A clinician's comfort with the techniques and interpretation of findings can assist with rapid diagnosis and initiation of appropriate treatment.

CLINICS CARE POINTS

- Office-based microscopy offers a point-of-care, inexpensive diagnostic tool that can be used for examination of vaginal discharge, skin scrapings, amniotic fluid ferning, urine sediment, and semen analysis when performed in a Clinical Laboratory Improvement Amendments of 1988–certified laboratory.

- Patients with symptoms of vaginitis, including vaginal discharge, odor, itching, pain, or redness, should undergo examination including microscopy; medical history alone is insufficient for diagnosis.

- Microscopy with application of Amsel criteria is the gold standard for diagnosis of bacterial vaginosis. If Amsel criteria are not met, no further testing or treatment is recommended.

- Wet prep and potassium hydroxide (KOH) examination have high specificity but poor sensitivity for diagnosing vaginal candidiasis and trichomoniasis. A negative examination may be followed up with further testing.

- With the addition of a centrifuge, office microscopy allows for urine sediment examination in the evaluation of acute kidney injury and chronic kidney disease and is often superior to automated urinalysis.

- Phase contrast microscopy is preferred over bright light microscopy for urine sediment.

- Urine sediment examination is particularly useful in distinguishing acute tubular necrosis from prerenal acute kidney injury, and hematuria originating from the lower urinary tract versus the glomerulus.

- Direct visualization with microscopy of scabies mites (using oil) or hyphae/pseudohyphae (using KOH) is the gold standard for diagnosis of scabies infestation or fungal skin infections, respectively.

- Disruption of corneal epithelium can be visualized using fluorescein and Wood's lamp; however, it must be performed in the appropriate context to avoid missing serious eye conditions requiring urgent evaluation and treatment by a specialist.

- When using a Wood's lamp to assist in the diagnosis of skin rashes or lesions, be sure to note the presence (or absence) of fluorescence, as well as its color and distribution for accurate interpretation.

DISCLOSURE

The authors have nothing to disclose.

REFERENCES

1. Centers for Disease Control & Prevention, Division of Laboratory Systems. Provider-Performed Microscopy Procedures: A Focus on Quality Practices. Educational Booklet. pages 1–92. Available at: https://www.cdc.gov/clia/docs/15_258020-A_Stang_PPMP_Booklet_FINAL.pdf.
2. Danby CS, Althouse AD, Hillier SL, et al. Nucleic Acid Amplification Testing Compared With Cultures, Gram Stain, and Microscopy in the Diagnosis of Vaginitis. J Low Genit Tract Dis 2021;25(1):76–80.
3. Vaginitis in Nonpregnant Patients: ACOG Practice Bulletin, Number 215. Obstet Gynecol 2020;135(1):e1–17.
4. Workowski KA, Bolan GA. Sexually transmitted diseases treatment guidelines, 2015. MMWR Recomm Rep 2015;64(Rr-03):1–137.
5. Kalia N, Singh J, Kaur M. Microbiota in vaginal health and pathogenesis of recurrent vulvovaginal infections: a critical review. Ann Clin Microbiol Antimicrob 2020;19(1):5.
6. Marie Abdallah MHAaWM. Vulvovaginitis and Cervicitis. In: John E, Bennett RD, Blaser MJ, editors. Mandell, Douglas, and Bennett's Principles and Practice of infectious diseases. 9th ed. ed. Elsevier, Inc; 2020. p. 1462–76.e1463.

7. Amsel R, Totten PA, Spiegel CA, et al. Nonspecific vaginitis. Diagnostic criteria and microbial and epidemiologic associations. Am J Med 1983;74(1):14–22.
8. Schwebke JR, Gaydos CA, Nyirjesy P, et al. Diagnostic Performance of a Molecular Test versus Clinician Assessment of Vaginitis. J Clin Microbiol 2018;56(6).
9. Newkirk GR. Wet Smear and Potassium Hydroxide Preparation. In: Fowler GC, editor. Pfenninger and Fowler's procedures for primary care. 4th ed. Philadelphia, PA: Elsevier; 2020. p. 829, 823.
10. Cavanaugh C, Perazella MA. Urine Sediment Examination in the Diagnosis and Management of Kidney Disease: Core Curriculum 2019. Am J Kidney Dis 2019; 73(2):258–72.
11. Becker GJ, Garigali G, Fogazzi GB. Advances in Urine Microscopy. Am J Kidney Dis 2016;67(6):954–64.
12. Perazella MA. The urine sediment as a biomarker of kidney disease. Am J Kidney Dis 2015;66(5):748–55.
13. Palsson R, Colona MR, Hoenig MP, et al. Assessment of Interobserver Reliability of Nephrologist Examination of Urine Sediment. JAMA Netw Open 2020;3(8): e2013959.
14. Fogazzi GB, Delanghe J. Microscopic examination of urine sediment: Phase contrast versus bright field. Clin Chim Acta Int J Clin Chem 2018;487:168–73.
15. Fogazzi, GB, Garigali, G. Urinalysis. In Comprehensive Clinical Nephrology, 6th Ed. Edinburgh: Elsevier.p. 39-52. Available at: https://www.clinicalkey.com/dura/browse/bookChapter/3-s2.0-C20160003765.
16. Trayes KP, Savage K, Studdiford JS. Annular Lesions: Diagnosis and Treatment. Am Fam Physician 2018;98(5):283–91.
17. Kliegman R, Stanton B, St. Geme JW III, et al. Arthropod bites and infestations. In: Nelson's textbook of pediatrics. Edition 21. Philadelphia, PA: Elsevier Inc.; 2020. p. 3568–76. Available at: https://www.clinicalkey.com/dura/browse/bookChapter/3-s2.0-C20161017121.
18. Havlickova B, Czaika VA, Friedrich M. Epidemiological trends in skin mycoses worldwide. Mycoses. 2008;51(Suppl 4):2–15.
19. Chosidow O. Clinical practices. Scabies. N Engl J Med 2006 Apr 20;354(16): 1718–27. https://doi.org/10.1056/NEJMcp052784.
20. Dinulos JGH. Superficial fungal infections. In: Habif's clinical dermatology: a color guide to diagnosis and therapy. 7th Ed. Edinburgh: Elsevier; 2021. p. 483–524. Available at: https://www.clinicalkey.com/dura/browse/bookChapter/3-s2.0-C20170014118.
21. Levitt JO, Levitt BH, Akhavan A, et al. The sensitivity and specificity of potassium hydroxide smear and fungal culture relative to clinical assessment in the evaluation of tinea pedis: a pooled analysis. Dermatol Res Pract 2010;2010:764843.
22. Hahm JE, Kim CW, Kim SS. The efficacy of a nested polymerase chain reaction in detecting the cytochrome c oxidase subunit 1 gene of Sarcoptes scabiei var. hominis for diagnosing scabies. Br J Dermatol 2018;179(4):889–95.
23. Walter B, Heukelbach J, Fengler G, et al. Comparison of Dermoscopy, Skin Scraping, and the Adhesive Tape Test for the Diagnosis of Scabies in a Resource-Poor Setting. Arch Dermatol 2011;147(4):468–73.
24. Buttaravoli PM, Leffler SM. Corneal Abrasions. In: Minor Emergencies. 3rd Edition. Philadelphia, PA: Elsevier/Saunders; 2012. p. 68–71. Available at: http://www.clinicalkey.com/dura/browse/bookChapter/3-s2.0-C20090622595.
25. Gebhard RE. Woods lamp examination. In: Pfenninger & Fowler's procedures for primary care. 4th edition. Philadelphia, PA: Elsevier; 2020. p. 213–5. Available at: https://www.clinicalkey.com/dura/browse/bookChapter/3-s2.0-C20150067557.

26. Wipperman JL, Dorsch JN. Evaluation and management of corneal abrasions. Am Fam Physician 2013;87(2):114–20.
27. Ahmed F, House RJ, Feldman BH. Corneal Abrasions and Corneal Foreign Bodies. Prim Care 2015;42(3):363–75.
28. McGwin G Jr, Xie A, Owsley C. Rate of Eye Injury in the United States. Arch Ophthalmol 2005;123(7):970–6.
29. Hooker EA, Faulkner WJ, Kelly LD, et al. Prospective study of the sensitivity of the Wood's lamp for common eye abnormalities. Emerg Med J 2019;36(3):159–62.
30. Wolff K, Johnson RA, Suurmond D, et al. Fitzpatrick's color atlas and synopsis of clinical dermatology. In: ed, editor. 5th ed. New York: McGraw-Hill Medical Pub. Division; 2005.
31. Al Aboud DM, Gossman W. Woods Light. In: StatPearls. Treasure Island (FL): StatPearls Publishing Copyright © 2020, StatPearls Publishing LLC; 2020.
32. Rui P, Okeyode T. National Ambulatory Medical Care Survey: 2016 National Summary Tables. Available at: https://www.cdc.gov/nchs/data/ahcd/namcs_summary/2016_namcs_web_tables.pdf. Accessed January 19, 2021.
33. Silverberg NB. The Epidemiology of Vitiligo. Curr Dermatol Rep 2015;4(1):36–43.
34. Chua RF, Pico J. Dermal Melanocytosis. In: StatPearls. Treasure Island (FL): StatPearls Publishing Copyright © 2020, StatPearls Publishing LLC; 2020.

Pediatric Office Procedures

Melanie H. Sanders, MD[a],*, Vasudha Jain, MD[b], Michael Malone, MD[b]

KEYWORDS

- Pediatric procedures • Umbilical granuloma • Polydactyly • Frenotomy
- Nursemaid's elbow • Hair tourniquet • Tympanometry

KEY POINTS

- When prepared with the appropriate knowledge of common pediatric problems, primary care physicians can easily perform procedures at the point of care.
- Although generally accepted approaches to common pediatric problems exist, there is a significant degree of debate and lack of consensus for many of the procedures discussed.
- More high-quality trials focused on patient-oriented outcomes are needed to define the standard of care.

INTRODUCTION

Evaluation of pediatric patients and performing relevant procedures is a necessary skill for the primary care physician. This can prove to be an intimidating task, however, because many common pediatric procedures lack clear consensus regarding techniques and robust data for patient-oriented outcomes. Few of the procedures detailed here have large, high-quality clinical trials, and many of the topics discussed need additional study. Despite these challenges, both patients and systems of care can benefit from addressing simple procedures at the point of care.

This article specifically discusses common pediatric procedures including umbilical granuloma chemocautery, frenotomy, suture ligation of type B postaxial polydactyly, reduction of nursemaid's elbow, hair tourniquet removal, and tympanometry. For each procedure, the required materials, indications and contraindications, procedural techniques, and other management options are reviewed.

UMBILICAL GRANULOMA CHEMOCAUTERY
Overview

Umbilical granulomas occur in approximately 1 in 500 neonates.[1–3] The umbilical cord stump gradually dries and typically separates by 7 to 15 days after birth. Delayed

---

[a] Department of Family Medicine, East Carolina University Brody School of Medicine, 101 Heart Drive, Mail Stop 654, Greenville, NC 27858, USA; [b] Tidelands Health Family Medicine Residency Program, 4320 Holmestown Road, Myrtle Beach, SC 29588, USA
* Corresponding author.
E-mail address: SANDERSME14@ECU.EDU

Prim Care Clin Office Pract 48 (2021) 707–728
https://doi.org/10.1016/j.pop.2021.07.010
0095-4543/21/© 2021 Elsevier Inc. All rights reserved.

separation may be due to infection or underlying immunodeficiencies.[1,4] Although the mechanism of granuloma formation is incompletely understood, it is hypothesized that an inflammatory process may trigger granuloma formation.[1] Granulomas are an overgrowth of granulation tissue, and are characteristically described as a small (<10 mm), moist, light pink mass at the center of the umbilicus[1,5] (**Fig. 1**).

It is important to note that other conditions can also present as an umbilical mass. **Table 1** reviews the differential diagnosis for umbilical granuloma.

Chemocauterization with silver nitrate is accepted as a conventional treatment for umbilical granuloma.[1,4] Other studies have explored alternative techniques that may be applied at home. This section will focus on this technique of chemocauterization with silver nitrate applied in the primary care clinic.

Required Equipment

Only a few materials are needed to complete chemocauterization of an umbilical granuloma. **Box 1** lists the recommended materials.

Indications

- Umbilical granuloma

Contraindications

- Signs of infection or omphalitis
- Strong suspicion that the umbilical mass is due to alternate pathology other than umbilical granuloma
- Allergy to silver nitrate

Procedure

1. Prep the umbilical area with alcohol pads or chlorhexidine swabs.
2. Dry the area with sterile sponge/gauze pads to avoid leakage onto normal tissue.
3. Apply petroleum jelly with a cotton tip swab to the surrounding skin to minimize the risk of burns to normal skin.
4. Gently grasp the umbilical granuloma with forceps (**Fig. 2**).
5. Apply silver nitrate stick to the entire granuloma, including the base, making sure to avoid contact with normal skin (**Fig. 3**).
6. Remove any excess silver nitrate with a clean cotton tip swab.

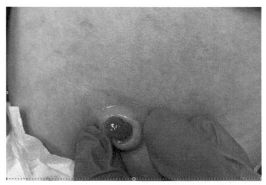

Fig. 1. Umbilical granuloma. (*Courtesy of* Shana Anton, MD of Tidelands Health, Myrtle Beach, SC and Melanie Sanders, MD, Greenville, NC.)

Table 1
Differential diagnosis for umbilical granuloma

Pathology Arising from Omphalomesenteric Duct Remnants (OMD, Also Called Vitelline Duct)	Pathology Arising from Urachal Remnants	Other Umbilical Masses or Abnormalities
• Meckel's diverticulum (most common 0.6%–4% of the population)[4] • Mucosal polyp • Umbilical enteric fistula (drains enteric contents) • Vitelline sinus • Vitelline cyst (rare)	• Urachal cyst (most common)[5] • Vesicoumbilical fistula (drains urine) • Urachal sinus • Diverticulum of bladder • Urachal polyp	• Umbilical hernia • Umbilical polyp (associated with an underlying OMD anomaly 30%–60% of cases)[4] • Adenomatous mass • Ectopic tissue (pancreatic or hepatic) • Dermoid or epidermoid cysts • Malignant tumors (teratoma, rhabdomyosarcoma, fibrous histiosarcoma) • Omphalitis

Data from Refs.[1,4–6]

7. Procedure may be repeated every 3 to 4 days if granuloma persists, for a maximum of 3 to 4 treatments.[1]

Complications

- Burns, skin discoloration, and ulcerations[2,4,6,7]
- Infection
- Failure to resolve, in which case referral for surgical excision is indicated[4,5]

Other Treatment Options

Other treatment options have been proposed to treat umbilical granulomas. Several small studies have evaluated salt application as a treatment option.[1,3,8–10] Although no significant complications have been noted (other than failure to resolve, in the case of umbilical polyps), this technique generally has been limited to use in developing countries or in cases in which no medical professional is available for silver nitrate application.[1,9]

Steroid application has also been evaluated as a potential treatment for umbilical granulomas. Studies evaluating steroid application using clobetasol propionate cream

Box 1
Recommended materials for chemocauterization of an umbilical granuloma

- Alcohol pads or chlorhexidine swabs for cleansing
- Sterile sponge/gauze
- Silver nitrate sticks (75% silver nitrate, 25% potassium nitrate)
- Petroleum jelly
- Cotton tip swab
- Forceps

Data from Karaguzel G, Aldemir H. Umbilical granuloma: Modern Understanding of Etiopathogenesis, Diagnosis and Management. J of Pediatr Neonatal Care. 2016;4(3):00136.

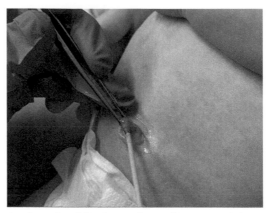

Fig. 2. Chemocauterization of umbilical granuloma. (*Courtesy of* Shana Anton, MD, Myrtle Beach, SC and Melanie Sanders, MD, Greenville, NC.)

(0.05%) were underpowered to demonstrate noninferiority to silver nitrate[2] or did not meet the standard for noninferiority.[11] These studies also noted common complications of steroid use including skin atrophy and hypopigmentation, which were reported as reversible.[2,11] Although it has been proposed that the short duration of treatment with topical clobetasol is not a significant risk for hypothalamic-pituitary-axis suppression, this has not been formally studied.[2,11,12]

Suture ligation, electrocautery, and cryosurgery have also been mentioned as possible treatment options.[1,6]

A referral for surgical excision is indicated if the granuloma fails to respond to conventional treatment.[1,5]

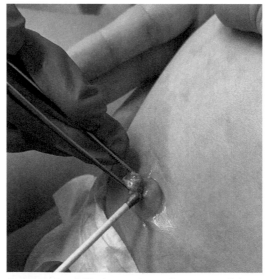

Fig. 3. Chemocauterization of umbilical granuloma. (*Courtesy of* Shana Anton, MD, Myrtle Beach, SC and Melanie Sanders, MD, Greenville, NC.)

Clinical Pearls

- Chemocauterization of umbilical granuloma is accepted as first-line treatment.
- Other pathology can present as umbilical masses in the neonate and should be considered on the differential diagnosis.
- Application of petroleum jelly to the surrounding skin and thoroughly drying the umbilical area can help prevent caustic burns to normal skin.
- If the umbilical granuloma does not respond to conventional treatment, a surgical referral is indicated to excise the mass and rule out other pathology.

SUTURE LIGATION OF POSTAXIAL POLYDACTYLY
Overview

There are many types of congenital hand deformities of variable complexity. Of these, postaxial polydactyly (also called ulnar polydactyly or supernumerary digit) is the most common[13,14] Temtamy and McKusic describe the 2 presentations of postaxial polydactyly as type A and type B.[14,15] Type A postaxial polydactyly is a fully formed supernumerary digit containing bony, ligamentous, and neural structures.[14,15] Type B postaxial polydactyly is a rudimentary structure consisting only of soft tissue, which is usually connected by a pedunculated stalk.[13–15] The connection point for type B can vary in size and may determine how the digit is managed (**Fig. 4**).

The total number of cases of postaxial polydactyly has been variably reported, but the condition appears to occur in approximately 4 of 10,000 live births.[13] Because type B postaxial polydactyly is typically inherited in an autosomal dominant pattern with variable penetrance, nearly 85% of cases have a positive family history.[15–17] African-American children are more commonly affected (1 in 143 live births) compared with Caucasian children (1 in 1339 live births).[15,18] Approximately, 70% to 75% of type B postaxial polydactyly cases are bilateral.[17,19]

Postaxial polydactyly can occur as an isolated finding or in conjunction with genetic syndromes.[15,19,20] Postaxial polydactyly without a family history should prompt a referral to a geneticist to evaluate for an underlying syndrome.[19]

Type A postaxial polydactyly requires referral for surgical intervention.[21] Management of type B postaxial polydactyly via suture ligation may be undertaken by the primary care physician. This technique is somewhat controversial because of potential complications and reports of more favorable results with fewer complications when

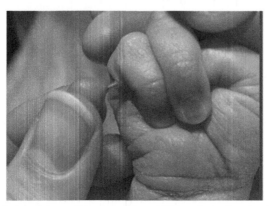

Fig. 4. Postaxial polydactyly type B, connection with a pedunculated stalk. (*Courtesy of* Allison Kuipers, MD, Charleston, SC.)

alternative surgical approaches are used.[13,15–17,19,22–24] A recent systematic review concluded that high-quality trials focused on patient-oriented outcomes are lacking, indicating the need for additional study regarding comparison of techniques to determine the optimal management of type B postaxial polydactyly.[13]

The procedure is described below. After suture ligation, the supernumerary digit will typically necrose and autoamputate within a period between 7 and 21 days (average 10 days).[15,23]

Required Equipment

Recommended materials for suture ligation of type B postaxial polydactyly include:

- 4-0 silk suture[16]
- Povidone iodine or chlorhexidine swabs for prepping the area
- Scissors

Indications

- Type B postaxial polydactyly with narrow base (pedunculated stalk ≤ 2 mm)[16,17,23] (**Fig. 5**)

Contraindications

- Type A postaxial polydactyly
  - If a bony structure is palpated on examination, an x-ray should be obtained before ligation is attempted.[19]
- Wide-based type B postaxial polydactyly (>2 mm)[16,17,23]
- Parental distress or lack of acceptance of the visual appearance and course of events with suture ligation

Procedure: Suture Ligation of Type B Postaxial Polydactyly

1. Cleanse and prepare the entire supernumerary digit and surrounding skin with povidone-iodine or chlorhexidine rinse.

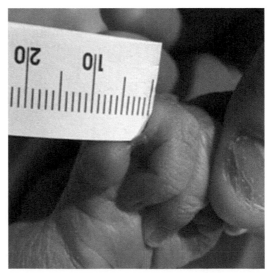

Fig. 5. Measurement of the base of the pedunculated stalk. (*Courtesy of* Allison Kuipers, MD, Charleston, SC.)

2. Position and tie the suture tightly at the base of the rudimentary digit, making 3 to 4 passes around the base of the digit and securing the knots tightly. Distal traction on the rudimentary digit is helpful to ensure that the ligature is placed at the most basal aspect of the digit. Clip the excess suture with scissors.
3. During the interim, the supernumerary digit will become discolored and necrotic. Often, the digit will autoamputate, but it may persist.
4. Reassess in approximately 7 to 10 days to ensure successful ligation. If remaining necrotic tissue is present, this may be removed with a pair of sharp scissors or can be monitored with frequent reassessment (**Fig. 6**).

Complications

A recent systematic review included a retrospective study that reported a complication rate of 23.5% with suture ligation and 3% in the surgical intervention group.[13] The potential complications of suture ligation of type B postaxial polydactyly are included in **Box 2**.

Other Treatment Options

Other techniques for the management of type B postaxial polydactyly require surgical referral. Surgical excision of the supernumerary digit has been studied both with topical anesthetic[22] and with local anesthetic using 0.5% lidocaine with epinephrine.[24,25] Surgical clips have also been used to treat this condition.[13,15,17] If parents elect surgical management, there is no concrete recommendation regarding the ideal timing. Recommendations vary from immediate excision during the newborn period to delayed excision under general anesthesia after 12 months of age.[15,19,24]

Clinical Pearls

- Type A postaxial polydactyly includes the presence of bony, ligamentous, and neural tissue elements, whereas the rudimentary structure of type B postaxial polydactyly includes only soft tissue.
- Suture ligation is an option for postaxial polydactyly, and appropriate counseling regarding potential complications and the appearance of the ligated digit will help ensure parents are well-informed.
- There is a lack of high-quality, patient-oriented evidence comparing various management strategies of type B postaxial polydactyly.

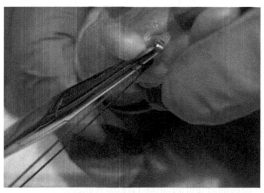

Fig. 6. Image showing suture at the base of postaxial polydactyly type B. This particular photo shows the supernumerary digit has also been clamped. (*Courtesy of* Allison Kuipers, MD, Charleston, SC.)

Box 2
Complications associated with suture ligation of type B postaxial polydactyly

- Neuroma (painful scar)
- Painful venous congestion
- Incomplete ligation (cosmetically unacceptable persistence of residual tissue)
- Cyst formation
- Infection
- Need for surgical revision

Data from Refs.[13,15–17,19,23]

Acknowledgments: Special thanks to Mia Amaya, MD, Associate Professor of Pediatrics and Medical Director of the Newborn Nursery at the Medical University of South Carolina for **Figs. 4–6**. Thank you also to Adam Ridley, MD and Victoria Sullivan, MD of the MUSC Family Medicine Residency Program, for contribution of additional postaxial polydactyly photographs.

FRENOTOMY
Overview

Ankyloglossia, also known as tongue-tie, is characterized by a short or thickened frenulum that restricts movement of the tongue. The estimated incidence of ankyloglossia has been variably reported, ranging from 0.02% to as high as 11% to 12%.[26,27] One study that examined the KIDS Database in the United States noted a substantial increase in the number of ankyloglossia cases from 1997 to 2012.[26] Male infants are more commonly affected.[26]

Several classification schemes exist; however, there is a lack of clear consensus regarding the diagnostic criteria for ankyloglossia.[28–30] A recent Clinical Consensus Statement from the American Academy of Otolaryngology—Head and Neck Surgery was unable to recommend a preferred diagnostic tool.[31] **Box 3** includes some of the diagnostic assessments for tongue tie.

Frequently described physical findings include restriction of tongue mobility, a "heart-shaped" tongue with crying, and dimpling of the tongue.[36] (**Fig. 7**. Photo of Lingual Frenulum. Photo Credit: Jill Aiken, MD and Katie Gagan, MD of Tidelands Health.)

Ankyloglossia may also have associated functional deficits in the infant that are of particular clinical relevance when deciding to proceed with frenotomy. These may

---

Box 3
Examples of diagnostic tools for ankyloglossia

- Coryllos system[32]
- Kotlow system[33]
- Hazelbaker Assessment Tool (HATLFF)[34]
- Neonatal Tongue Screening Test from the Lingual Frenulum Protocol for Infants (LFPI)[35]
- Bristol Tongue Assessment Tool (BTAT)[28]

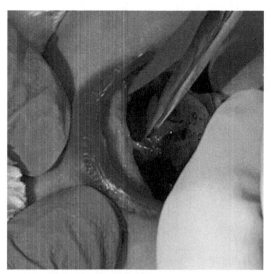

Fig. 7. Lingual frenulum. (*Courtesy of* Jill Aiken, MD, Myrtle Beach, SC and Katie Gagan, MD, Myrtle Beach, SC.)

affect breastfeeding, with problems such as poor latch and extended feeding duration, which can lead to failure to thrive or distressing maternal complications, such as nipple pain or breast engorgement.[30,32,36] In addition, there are some concerns that persistent ankyloglossia may have speech and additional oral motor concerns in older children.[5] Both AHRQ and a 2015 systematic review found that current data are insufficient to assess effects of frenotomy for outcomes other than breastfeeding.[30,37]

Frenotomy improves maternal nipple pain in the short term but does not produce a consistent improvement in infant breastfeeding.[27,31]

Owing to lack of consensus regarding diagnosis, and lack of consistent results in breastfeeding and long-term outcomes, the management of ankyloglossia remains controversial.[30,31]

Required Equipment

Suggested Equipment for Frenotomy
- Oral sucrose solution (24%)
- Grooved retractor
- Straight clamp
- Scissors
- Gauze
- Silver nitrate may be used for hemostasis, if needed

Indications

Potential indications for frenotomy include:[30]

- Poor feeding with infant complications:
  - Failure to thrive
  - Poor weight gain
- Poor feeding with maternal concerns:
  - Breast pain
  - Inadequate milk extraction leading to poor supply

- ○ Breast engorgement
- ○ Nipple/breast pain

Frenotomy is not recommended to prevent possible future speech or feeding problems in infants with minimal to no tongue restriction.[31]

Contraindications

Contraindications to frenotomy include[31]:

- Other more likely causes of feeding difficulty other than ankyloglossia, such as craniofacial abnormalities, nasal or airway obstruction
- Deformities affecting the jaw that may result in airway obstruction after frenotomy, including retrognathia and micrognathia
- Neuromuscular disorders
- Hypotonia
- Coagulopathy

Procedure

1. Oral sucrose may be administered before the procedure.[31,36]
2. Swaddle the child to restrict the movement of the arms. After placing the child in position, have an assistant hold the infant's head.
3. Isolate the lingual frenulum with a grooved retractor (**Fig. 8**).
4. Crush the frenulum tissue with the straight clamp to aid in hemostasis.[38]
5. Cut the thin attachment of the frenulum, taking care to not extend into the muscle (**Fig. 9**).
6. Place digital pressure on the area with gauze for several seconds. If difficulty achieving hemostasis is encountered, silver nitrate may be used to cauterize any bleeding areas.
7. The infant may feed immediately after the procedure.

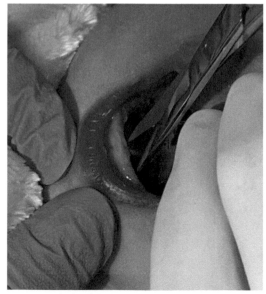

Fig. 8. Isolation of the lingual frenulum with a grooved retractor. (*Courtesy of* Jill Aiken, MD, Myrtle Beach, SC and Katie Gagan, MD, Myrtle Beach, SC.)

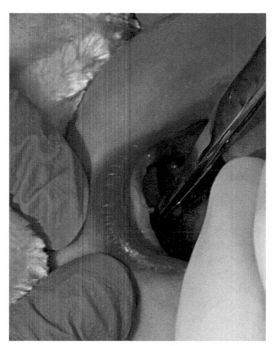

Fig. 9. Cut the thin attachment of the lingual frenulum, but avoid extending the cut into the muscle. (*Courtesy of* Jill Aiken, MD, Myrtle Beach, SC and Katie Gagan, MD, Myrtle Beach, SC.)

Topical and local anesthetic agents are not recommended.[31]

Complications

Complication rates for frenotomy are low; however, there is moderate strength of evidence for minimal and short-lived bleeding postprocedure.[30] In rare cases, more significant bleeding resulting in hemorrhagic shock has been reported, although these cases occurred after frenotomy by untrained personnel[39] or in older children.[28]

Additional complications may include damage to surrounding structures (tongue, lip, salivary ducts, lingual nerve), infection, recurrence, oral aversion, scarring, and failure to improve breastfeeding.[31,36,40]

Additional case reports resulted in airway compromise after frenotomy in infants with Pierre Robin sequence.[41]

Other Options

Frenotomy has been performed with laser or electrocautery or with more complex surgical techniques. There is insufficient evidence that one technique is superior to the others.[31]

Clinical Pearls

- Frenotomy is a highly debated topic, and lack of consensus regarding diagnosis and management creates challenges for the primary care physician.
- Indications for frenotomy include breastfeeding difficulties affecting either the mother or the child.

- Other conditions that can cause feeding difficulties and should be ruled out before proceeding with frenotomy.
- Frenotomy may result in improvement in nipple pain and improved maternal reports of breastfeeding efficacy, but evidence for consistent improvement in infant breastfeeding is lacking and requires further study.

Introduction

Hair tourniquet syndrome (HTS) occurs when a strand of hair becomes tightly wrapped around a body part, usually a digit in an infant. It is poorly recognized in the pediatric population, and prompt recognition is critical. HTS should be suspected in irritable children, with focused examination to look for signs of strangulation of an appendage. Magnification is often needed for adequate visualization of the hair. HTS can lead to ischemic gangrene and autoamputation if not recognized and treated early.[42,43] The hair or fiber wrapped around an appendage causes decreased venous drainage, which leads to edema. The swelling can result in pressure on the end arteries of the digits leading to tissue necrosis and later to autoamputation. The affected digit may appear swollen or erythematous.[44] Hair tourniquets can involve multiple appendages including toes, fingers, and even genitalia.[44] The majority of cases are in infants 2 months of age or younger.[44]

Procedure
Indications
- Superficial hair tourniquet.
Contraindications
- Tissue necrosis or ischemia noted; consult specialty services.[45]
Approach
- Before the procedure, make sure you have inspected the affected arm for any deformities.
- Place the patient in a well-lit area and make sure the patient is neurovascularly intact.[45]
- Place patient's affected appendage in a comfortable position and ask the caregiver for support.[46]
- Depilatory cream on intact skin for 3 to 6 minutes can help assist in hair breakdown.[46,47]
1. The Cut Method (in-office)[46]
   a. Use EMLA cream or a topical anesthetic to the area
   b. Use curved hemostats or blunt probes to lift hair away from appendage
   c. Use scissors to carefully cut the hair to relieve the strangulation
2. The Unwind Method[46]
   a. Use EMLA cream or a topical anesthetic to the area
   b. Use curved hemostats or blunt probes to lift hair away and cut a portion of the hair
   c. Carefully unwind the hair to relieve pressure from the appendage
3. The Surgical Method should be used for a deeper strangulation and should be performed by a specialist such as plastic surgeon, pediatric surgeon, urologist, or gynecologist, depending on the area of strangulation.

Recovery

Patients should feel improvement almost immediately, though total improvement can take up to 1 week. A neurovascular examination should be performed after completion of the procedure. Usually, a course of antibiotics, such as amoxicillin, is indicated, especially after surgical removal of the strangulation.[45] On superficial strangulation cases, the use of topical antibiotic cream may be helpful. NSAIDs or acetaminophen can be used for pain reduction if needed. Patients should be re-evaluated within 24 hours to 1 week.[46]

Follow-up with plastic surgeon, pediatric surgeon, urologist, or gynecologist might be necessary depending on the level of injury or affected appendage.[46]

Summary

HTS is rare and mostly affects infants with mothers experiencing telogen effluvium. The areas that are most often affected include toes, fingers, genitalia (ie, penis, vulva, clitoris), but can also affect ear lobes and nipples. Most often this is accidental, but child abuse must still be considered.[46] Depending on the degree and location of strangulation, surgical methods may be considered. Surgical methods should be performed by a specialist to preserve the soft tissue affected.[46] Close follow-up is necessary and postoperative care with oral or topical antibiotics is recommended.[47]

Pearls
- Suspect HTS in pediatric patients with swollen appendages with apparent strangulation.
- Early diagnosis and management is required to avoid tissue necrosis and autoamputation.
- If signs of neurovascular injury or unsuccessful office methods, urgent referral to a surgical specialist is indicated.
- Most often after removal of the strangulation, the edema in the affected appendage resolves over time.

NURSEMAID'S ELBOW
Introduction

Nursemaid's elbow, also known as radial head subluxation or a pulled elbow, is a common complaint in the pediatric population. It can occur in children from 2 months of age to those up to 10 to 11 years old. Most commonly, the condition occurs in children aged 5 years and younger secondary to weaker ligaments.[48] Nursemaid's elbow often occurs as a result of a "pull injury" by an adult or a taller individual where there is sudden pulling or tugging of the extended arm. The mechanism of injury may also be a fall. Sudden longitudinal traction on the extended arm causes subluxation of the radial head by pulling the radial head through the annular ligament. Commonly, the child has acute pain and refuses to use the arm. Intervention involves reduction using the supination-flexion method or the hyperpronation method. The purpose of the interventions is to reposition the radial head within the annular ligament.[49,50] It is unclear which maneuver is superior.[51]

Diagnosis

The diagnosis is based on clinical suspicion. The typical presentation is when a child suddenly cries out in pain and refuses to move his/her arm after a pulling incident.[49] Often a "click" is heard at the time of injury. Patients usually present with the arm in a slightly flexed position close to the body and with the forearm in pronation. They may also present with the arm held to the side in full extension. Often there is tenderness with palpation over the anterolateral aspect of the radial head without any obvious swelling or deformity. Radiographic imaging is less helpful in establishing the diagnosis.[48,50]

Anatomy

The injury is located at the anterolateral aspect of the elbow as the radial head is pulled through the annular ligament. Tenderness along the radial head is common. The patient in **Fig. 11** is holding the arm in typical fashion with slight flexion and with the forearm pronated (**Fig. 10**).

Procedure
  Indications
  • Radial head subluxation
  Contraindications
  • Suspected fracture or inconsistent history
Approach
• Before the procedure, be sure to inspect the affected arm for any deformities and examine the entire arm from clavicle to fingers.
• Place patient in a comfortable position in caretaker's lap facing the clinician.
• Place patient with affected arm facing the clinician.

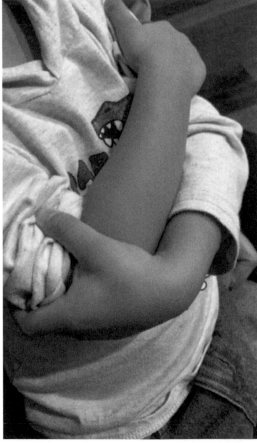

Fig. 10. Typical positioning of the affected arm. (*Courtesy of* Vasudha Jain, MD, Myrtle Beach, SC.)

- To reduce anxiety, approach patient at eye level and calmly distract attention away from the affected arm.

Hyperpronation Method

- Place the palm of your hand under the dorsal portion of the elbow with the elbow in 90° flexion.
- Apply pressure using your thumb at the anterolateral aspect of the elbow, over the radial head, and place your other palm on the ventral aspect of the child's forearm.
- Internally rotate (or pronate) the forearm while applying pressure and listen for a "click" or a "pop" (**Fig. 11**).

Supination-Flexion Method

- Place the palm of your hand under the elbow similar to the hyperpronation method.
- Grip the palmar aspect of the child's wrist while applying gentle traction.
- While applying traction, externally rotate (or supinate) the patient's wrist and fully flex the elbow and listen for a "click" or "pop" (**Fig. 12**).

Recovery

Patient should feel improvement almost immediately and will start to move their affected arm within 5 to 10 minutes.[49] No other intervention is required. Return instructions should be given to the caretaker.

Management

Radial head subluxation is usually improved with reduction alone. It does not require any immobilization, follow-up imaging, or activity restrictions. After successful reduction, follow-up is not necessary. An orthopedic evaluation is not necessary. NSAIDs or acetaminophen can be used for pain reduction.

Outcomes

If there are multiple unsuccessful attempts, x-ray imaging is warranted. If imaging is normal, the patient should be placed in a sling and outpatient follow-up should be arranged. If fracture is suspected, x-ray imaging should be obtained and pediatric orthopedic follow-up should be arranged. Children with a history of radial head subluxation

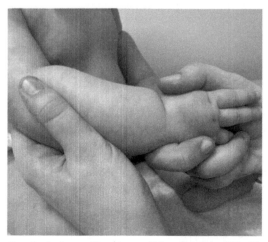

Fig. 11. Hyperpronation technique. (*Courtesy of* Vasudha Jain, MD, Myrtle Beach, SC.)

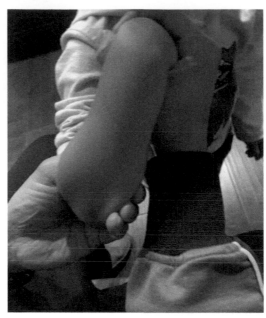

Fig. 12. Supination flexion method. (*Courtesy of* Vasudha Jain, MD, Myrtle Beach, SC.)

will have a higher risk of future subluxation, and caretakers should avoid forcefully pulling on the affected arm.[49]

Summary

Radial head subluxation, or nursemaid's elbow, is usually caused by a pulling injury from a taller individual and occurs in children younger than 5 years due to a weaker annular ligament. It is a clinical diagnosis and imaging is not needed or helpful for diagnosis. If there are multiple unsuccessful attempts at reduction, x-ray imaging is warranted to rule out a fracture. There are 2 common techniques of reduction: the hyperpronation method and the supination-flexion method. A Cochrane review was unable to find high-quality evidence to recommend one method over the other but did have low-level evidence that concluded the hyperpronation method might have lower first-time failure rates.[48]

Pearls

- Radial head subluxation, also known as nursemaid's elbow, is usually caused by a pulling injury by a taller individual on a straight arm.
- Patients present with acute pain with refusal to move the affected arm.
- The affected arm is usually held in flexion and pronation or is hanging straight close to the body.
- Radiographic imaging is not needed for diagnosis.
- Hyperpronation method and supination-flexion method are the most commonly used techniques.
- Pain is resolved almost immediately, and the patient might take 5 to 10 minutes to use the arm normally.
- Obtain x-ray imaging if there are multiple failed attempts at reduction or a fracture is suspected.

TYMPANOMETRY
Introduction

Tympanometry is an objective measure of the changes in acoustic impedance of the middle ear in response to variable changes in pressure. In combination with history and physical examination, it provides useful information about the presence of fluid in the middle ear, mobility of the middle ear system, and ear canal volume. It can be used in combination with patient history and examination findings, such as a bulging tympanic membrane (TM), for the evaluation of otitis media, eustachian tube dysfunction, and TM perforation. Studies combining tympanometry with clinical signs and symptoms have shown a sensitivity of 90% and a specificity of 75% in diagnosing otitis media with effusion.[52] Tympanometry is not reliable in infants younger than 7 months because of the high compliance of infant's ear canals.[53]

Complications/Risks of the Procedure

There are no significant risks related to the tympanometry test.

How to Perform the Procedure

Before inserting the tympanometer, the external ear canal should be assessed with an otoscope to ensure there is no cerumen or foreign object obstructing the external ear canal. Next, the tympanometer is placed snugly in the ear canal. A sound stimulus generator transmits acoustic energy into the canal while a vacuum pump introduces positive and negative pressures into the ear canal. A microphone in the instrument detects returning sound energy to produce a tympanogram based on the results.[53] The point of maximum compliance of the TM correlates with the air pressure in the middle ear. Patients should not speak or swallow during the test, as this lowers the accuracy of the test. Several measurements are often needed for optimal results, but the total procedural time is typically 2 to 3 minutes.

RESULTS OF TYMPANOMETRY

A tympanometry report, or tympanogram, describes the ear canal volume, middle ear pressure, and the peak compliance. Tympanogram results can be grouped into 5 categories:[53,54] (**Fig. 13**)

Type A: Normal tympanogram (see **Fig. 13**)

The type A tympanogram has a normal maximum height that occurs at a pressure close to zero, and the curve is symmetric. A type A tracing indicates normal tympanometry test results and denotes no fluid in the middle ear, normal compliance of the TM, normal middle ear pressure, and normal movement of the ossicles and TM.

Type B: Abnormal tympanogram: a flat line with no identifiable peak (see **Fig. 13**)

Of all the tympanogram tracings, a type B finding best predicts middle ear dysfunction or abnormality. There at 2 circumstances that may cause this result:[53]

1. Otitis media with fluid or pus behind the TM, which allows minimal or no mobility of the TM. In this situation, a straight flat line overlays the X-axis (ear canal volume is normal).
2. Ruptured TMs, which results in a flat line parallel to and above the x-axis (higher ear canal volume).

Other causes for type B tracings are TM scarring causing immobility, tympanosclerosis, cholesteatoma, or a middle ear tumor.[53]

Type C: Likely abnormal tympanogram: pressure is negative, correlating with a retracted TM (see **Fig. 13**)

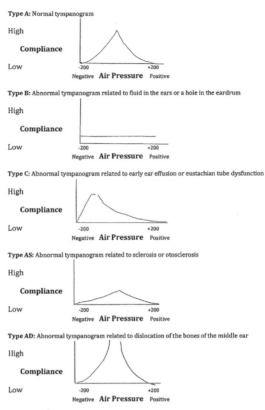

Fig. 13. Tympanogram results.

Type C tympanograms with slight to moderately negative pressure can be considered a normal variant, whereas highly negative pressure is typically considered abnormal.[55] This result can be suggestive of an ear effusion or eustachian tube dysfunction. A type C curve may be clinically useful when correlated with other findings but is not highly predictive for diagnosing middle ear disorders in isolation.[56]

Type AS: Abnormal tympanogram: reduced peak height due to a less compliant middle ear (see **Fig. 13**)

The low compliance of a type AS tympanogram can be related to sclerosis or otosclerosis.[57]

Type AD: Abnormal tympanogram: extremely high peak height that may be off the tracing with high compliance due to hypermobility (see **Fig. 13**)

A type AD result can be caused by dislocation of the ossicles or from a partially healed TM perforation that is thin and highly compliant.[53]

SUMMARY OF KEY CLINICAL POINTS

Tympanometry provides a method to diagnose and monitor middle ear pathology.

Tympanometry is most accurate when used in combination with history, physical examination, and/or other test results.

There are 5 main categories of tympanogram results.

A type A tympanogram is a normal result suggesting no significant middle ear dysfunction.

A type B finding best predicts a middle ear abnormality.

CLINICS CARE POINTS

- Once significant (but exceptionally uncommon) pathology is excluded, chemocautery of umbilical granuloma is a quick, simple, and low-risk office procedure.

- In-office suture ligation of a supernumerary digit (postaxial polydactyly) is only appropriate for rudimentary soft tissue structures that do not contain bony, ligamentous, or neural components.

- The primary indication for neonatal lingual frenotomy is breastfeeding difficulty resulting from restricted tongue movement that also limits infant weight gain or causes maternal breast concerns.

- Hair tourniquet syndrome is rare but can cause substantial physical complications; a high index of suspicion is appropriate when evaluating an irritable infant.

- Radial head subluxation is a clinical diagnosis and does not require imaging unless the mechanism of injury is inconsistent with nursemaid's elbow or multiple attempts at reduction are unsuccessful.

- Tympanometry compliments the diagnostic examination and offers rapid, objective verification of middle ear pathology.

DISCLOSURE

The authors have nothing to disclose.

REFERENCES

1. Karaguzel G, Aldemir H. Umbilical granuloma: Modern Understanding of Etiopathogenesis, Diagnosis and Management. J Pediatr Neonatal Care 2016;4(3): 00136.
2. Brødsgaard A, Nielsen T, Mølgaard U, et al. Treating umbilical granuloma with topical clobetasol propionate cream at home is as effective as treating it with topical silver nitrate in the clinic. Acta Paediatr 2015;104:174-7.
3. Haftu H, Gebremichael TG, Kebedom AG. Salt Treatment for Umbilical Granuloma – An Effective, Cheap, and Available Alternative Treatment Option: Case Report. Pediatr Health Med Ther 2020;11:393-7. https://doi.org/10.2147/PHMT. S269114.
4. Muniraman H, Sardesai T, Sardesai S. Disorders of the umbilical cord. Pediatr Rev 2018;39:332-41.
5. O'Donnell KA, Glick PL, Caty MG. Pediatric umbilical probems. Pediatr Clin North Am 1998;45(4):791-9.
6. Lotan G, Klin B, Efrati Y. Double-ligature: a treatment for pedunculated umbilical granulomas in children. Am Fam Physician 2002;65(10):2067-8.
7. Silver-nitrate: Skin burns: 2 case reports. React Weekly 2018;4:235.
8. Bagadia J, Jaiswal S, Bhalala KB, et al. Pinch of salt: A modified technique to treat umbilical granuloma. Pediatr Dermatol 2019;36:561-3.
9. Haftu H, Bitew H, Gebrekidan A, et al. The Outcome of Salt Treatment for Umbilical Granuloma: A Systematic Review. Patient Prefer Adherence 2020;14: 2085-92.

10. Lees D, Chua YW, Gilla A. Seasoning your umbilical granuloma: Steroid glaze or a pinch of salt? J Paediatr Child Health 2019;55(7):857–9.
11. Ogawa C, Sato Y, Suzuki C, et al. Treatment with silver nitrate versus topical steroid treatment for umbilical granuloma: A non-inferiority randomized control trial. PLoS One 2018;13:e0192688.
12. Aydin M, Orman A, Deveci U, et al. Topical clobetasol propionate may not be safe for treating umbilical granuloma in infants. Acta Paediatr 2015;104:e49.
13. Chopan M, Sayadi L, Chim H, et al. To tie or not to tie: a systematic review of postaxial polydactyly and outcomes of suture ligation versus surgical excision. Hand (N Y). 2020;15(3):303–10.
14. Pino Paula, Zlotolow Dan, Kozin Scott. What's New in Congenital Hand Surgery. J Pediatr Orthop 2020;40(8):e753–60.
15. Wessel Lauren, Daluiski Aaron, Trehan Samir. Polydactyly a review and update of a common congenital hand difference. Curr Opin Pediatr 2020;32(1):120–4.
16. Mullick S, Borschel GH. A Selective Approach to Treatment of Ulnar Polydactyly: Preventing Painful Neuroma and Incomplete Excision. Pediatr Dermatol 2010;27: 39–42.
17. Rathjen NA, Rogers TS, Garigan TP, et al. Management of Postaxial Polydactyly in the Neonatal Unit. J Am Osteopath Assoc 2017;117(11):719–21.
18. Watson BT, Hennrikus WL. Postaxial type-B polydactyly. Prevalence and treatment. J Bone Joint Surg Am 1997;79(1):65–8.
19. Comer GC, Potter M, Ladd AL. Polydactyly of the Hand. J Am Acad Orthop Surg 2018;26(3):75–82.
20. Ahmed H, Akbari H, Emami A, et al. Genetic Overview of Syndactyly and Polydactyly. Plast Reconstr Surg Glob Open 2017;5(11):e1549.
21. Kozin S, Zlotolow D. Common Pediatric Congenital Conditions of the Hand. Plast Reconstr Surg 2015;136(2):241e–57e.
22. Katz K, Linder N. Postaxial Type B Polydactyly Treated by Excision in the Neonatal Nursery. J Pediatr Orthop 2011;31(4):448–9.
23. Patillo D, Rayan GM. Complications of suture ligation ablation for ulnar polydactyly: a report of two cases. Hand (N Y). 2011;6(1):102–5.
24. Carpenter CL, Cuellar TA, Friel MT. Office-Based Post-Axial Polydactyly Excision in Neonates, Infants, and Children. Plast Reconstr Surg 2016;137(2):564–8.
25. Mantilla-Rivas E, Tan P, Zajac J, et al. Is Epinephrine Safe for Infant Digit Excision? A Retrospective Review of 402 Polydactyly Excisions in Patients Younger than 6 Months. Plast Reconstr Surg 2019;144(1):149–54.
26. Walsh J, Links A, Boss E, et al. Ankyloglossia and Lingual Frenotomy: National Trends in Inpatient Diagnosis and Management in the United States, 1997-2012. Otolaryngol Head Neck Surg 2017;156(4):735–40.
27. O'Shea, Joyce E, Foster, et al. Frenotomy for tongue-tie in newborn infants. Cochrane Database Syst Rev 2017;(3). Available from EBM Reviews - Cochrane Database of Systematic Reviews at: http://ovidsp.ovid.com/ovidweb.cgi?T=JS&PAGE=reference&D=coch&NEWS=N&AN=00075320-100000000-09466. Accessed December 28, 2020.
28. Walsh J, McKenna Benoit M. Ankyloglossia and Other Oral Ties. Otolaryngol Clin North Am 2019;52(5):795–811.
29. Unger C, Chetwynd E, Costello R. Ankyloglossia Identification, Diagnosis, and Frenotomy: A Qualitative Study of Community Referral Pathways. J Hum lactation 2020;36(3):519–27.
30. Francis DO, Chinnadurai S, Morad A, et al. Treatments for ankyloglossia and ankyloglossia with Concomitant lip-tie. Comparative Effectiveness review No. 149.

(Prepared by the Vanderbilt evidence-based Practice center under Contract No. 290-2012-00009-I.) AHRQ Publication No. 15-EHC011-EF. Rockville (MD): Agency for Healthcare Research and Quality; 2015. Available at: www. effectivehealthcare.ahrq.gov/reports/final.cfm.

31. Messner AH, Walsh J, Rosenfeld RM, et al. Clinical Consensus Statement: Ankyloglossia in Children. Otolaryngol Head Neck Surg 2020;162(5):597–611.
32. Coryllos E, Genna C, Salloum AC. Congenital tongue-tie and its impact on breast-feeding. Am Acad Pediatr Section Breastfeed 2004;1–6.
33. Kotlow LA. Ankyloglossia (tongue tie): a diagnostic and treatment quandry. Quintessence Int 1999;30(4):259–62.
34. Amir LH, James JP, Donath SM. Reliability of the hazelbaker assessment tool for lingual frenulum function. Int Breastfeed J 2006;1(1):3.
35. Campanha SMA, Martinelli RL de C, Palhares DB. Association between ankyloglossia and breastfeeding. CoDAS 2019;31(1):e20170264.
36. Walsh J, Tunkel D. Diagnosis and Treatment of Ankyloglossia in Newborns and Infants: A Review. JAMA Otolaryngol Head Neck Surg 2017;143(10):1032–9.
37. Chinnadurai S, Francis DO, Richard A, et al. Treatment of Ankyloglossia for Reasons Other Than Breastfeeding: A Systematic Review. Pediatrics 2015;135(6): e1467–74.
38. Buryk M, Bloom D, Shope T. Efficacy of neonatal release of ankyloglossia: a randomized trial. Pediatrics 2011;128(2):280–8.
39. Opara PI, Gabriel-Job N, Opara KO. Neonates presenting with severe complications of frenotomy: a case series. J Med Case Rep 2012;6:77.
40. Brookes A, Bowley DM. Tongue tie: The evidence for frenotomy. Early Hum Dev 2014;90:765–8.
41. Genther DJ, Skinner ML, Bailey PJ, et al. Airway obstruction after lingual freulectomy in two infants with Pierre-Robin sequence. Int J Pediatr Otorhinolaryngol 2015;79(9):1592–4.
42. Sivathasan N, Vijayarajan L. Hair-thread tourniquet syndrome: a case report and literature review. Case Rep Med 2012;2012:171368.
43. Baloch N, Atif M, Rashid RH, et al. Toe-tourniquet syndrome: A rare potentially devastating entity. Malays Orthop J 2015;9(3):55–7.
44. Cevik Y, Kavalci C. Hair tourniquet syndrome. Ann Saudi Med 2010;30(5):416–7.
45. Dunphy L, Verma Y, Morhij R, et al. Hair thread tourniquet syndrome in a male infant: a rare surgical emergency. BMJ Case Rep 2017;2017. bcr2017221002.
46. Alruwaili N, Alshehri HA, Halimeh B. Hair tourniquet syndrome: Successful management with a painless technique. Int J Pediatr Adolesc Med 2015;2(1):34–7.
47. Aslantürk O, Özbey R, Yılmaz Ö, et al. Hair tourniquet syndrome of toes and fingers in infants. Acta Orthop Traumatol Turc 2019;53(4):306–9.
48. Krul M, van der Wouden JC, Kruithof EJ, et al. Manipulative interventions for reducing pulled elbow in young children. Cochrane Database Syst Rev 2017;(7):CD007759. Accessed January 19, 2021.
49. Cornelius AP, Avery LT. Radial head subluxation (nursemaid's elbow) reduction. In: Mayeaux EJ, editor. The essential guide to primary care procedures. 2nd edition. Philadelphia, PA: Wolters Kluwer; 2015. p. 110–3.
50. Salter RB, Zaltz C. Anatomic investigations of the mechanism of injury and pathologic anatomy of "pulled elbow" in young children. Clin Orthop Relat Res 1971; 77:134–43.
51. McDonald J, Whitelaw C, Goldsmith LJ. Radial Head Subluxation: Comparing Two Methods of Reduction. Acad Emerg Med 1999;6:715–8.

52. Johansen EC, Lildholdt T, Damsbo N, et al. Tympanometry for diagnosis and treatment of otitis media in general practice. Fam Pract 2000;17:317–22.
53. Onusko E. Tympanometry. Am Fam Physician 2004;70(9):1713–20.
54. Margolis RH, Hunter LL. Tympanometry: basic principles and clinical applications. In: Musiek FE, Rintelmann WF, editors. Contemporary perspectives in hearing assessment. Boston: Allyn and Bacon; 1999. p. 89–130.
55. Engel J, Anteunis L, Chenault M, et al. Otoscopic findings in relation to tympanometry during infancy. Eur Arch Otorhinolaryngol 2000;257:366–71.
56. Brookhouser PE. Use of tympanometry in office practice for diagnosis of otitis media. Pediatr Infect Dis J 1998;17:544–51.
57. Pensak M. Otosclerosis. In: Tami TA, editor. Otolaryngology: a case study approach. New York: Thieme; 1998. p. 21.

UNITED STATES POSTAL SERVICE®

Statement of Ownership, Management, and Circulation
(All Periodicals Publications Except Requester Publications)

1. Publication Title: PRIMARY CARE: CLINICS IN OFFICE PRACTICE

2. Publication Number: 044 – 690

3. Filing Date: 9/18/2021

4. Issue Frequency: MAR, JUN, SEP, DEC

5. Number of Issues Published Annually: 4

6. Annual Subscription Price: $261.00

7. Complete Mailing Address of Known Office of Publication *(Not printer) (Street, city, county, state, and ZIP+4®)*
ELSEVIER INC.
230 Park Avenue, Suite 800
New York, NY 10169

Contact Person: Malathi Samayan
Telephone *(Include area code)*: 91-44-4299-4507

8. Complete Mailing Address of Headquarters or General Business Office of Publisher *(Not printer)*
ELSEVIER INC.
230 Park Avenue, Suite 800
New York, NY 10169

9. Full Names and Complete Mailing Addresses of Publisher, Editor, and Managing Editor *(Do not leave blank)*

Publisher *(Name and complete mailing address)*
DOLORES MELON ELSEVIER INC.
1600 JOHN F KENNEDY BLVD. SUITE 1800
PHILADELPHIA, PA 19103-2899

Editor *(Name and complete mailing address)*
KATERINA HEIDHAUSEN, ELSEVIER INC.
1600 JOHN F KENNEDY BLVD. SUITE 1800
PHILADELPHIA, PA 19103-2899

Managing Editor *(Name and complete mailing address)*
PATRICK MANLEY, ELSEVIER INC.
1600 JOHN F KENNEDY BLVD. SUITE 1800
PHILADELPHIA, PA 19103-2899

10. Owner *(Do not leave blank. If the publication is owned by a corporation, give the name and address of the corporation immediately followed by the names and addresses of all stockholders owning or holding 1 percent or more of the total amount of stock. If not owned by a corporation, give the names and addresses of the individual owners. If owned by a partnership or other unincorporated firm, give its name and address as well as those of each individual owner. If the publication is published by a nonprofit organization, give its name and address.)*

Full Name	Complete Mailing Address
WHOLLY OWNED SUBSIDIARY OF REED/ELSEVIER, US HOLDINGS	1600 JOHN F KENNEDY BLVD. SUITE 1800 PHILADELPHIA, PA 19103-2899

11. Known Bondholders, Mortgagees, and Other Security Holders Owning or Holding 1 Percent or More of Total Amount of Bonds, Mortgages, or Other Securities. If none, check box ▶ ☐ None

Full Name	Complete Mailing Address
N/A	

12. Tax Status *(For completion by nonprofit organizations authorized to mail at nonprofit rates) (Check one)*
The purpose, function, and nonprofit status of this organization and the exempt status for federal income tax purposes:
☒ Has Not Changed During Preceding 12 Months
☐ Has Changed During Preceding 12 Months *(Publisher must submit explanation of change with this statement)*

PS Form **3526**, July 2014 [Page 1 of 4 *(see instructions page 4)*] PSN: 7530-01-000-9931   PRIVACY NOTICE: See our privacy policy on www.usps.com

---

13. Publication Title: PRIMARY CARE: CLINICS IN OFFICE PRACTICE

14. Issue Date for Circulation Data Below: JULY 2021

15. Extent and Nature of Circulation

			Average No. Copies Each Issue During Preceding 12 Months	No. Copies of Single Issue Published Nearest to Filing Date
a. Total Number of Copies *(Net press run)*			88	67
b. Paid Circulation *(By Mail and Outside the Mail)*	(1)	Mailed Outside-County Paid Subscriptions Stated on PS Form 3541 (Include paid distribution above nominal rate, advertiser's proof copies, and exchange copies)	42	35
	(2)	Mailed In-County Paid Subscriptions Stated on PS Form 3541 (Include paid distribution above nominal rate, advertiser's proof copies, and exchange copies)	0	0
	(3)	Paid Distribution Outside the Mails Including Sales Through Dealers and Carriers, Street Vendors, Counter Sales, and Other Paid Distribution Outside USPS®	14	8
	(4)	Paid Distribution by Other Classes of Mail Through the USPS (e.g. First-Class Mail®)	0	0
c. Total Paid Distribution *(Sum of 15b (1), (2), (3), and (4))*		▶	56	43
d. Free or Nominal Rate Distribution *(By Mail and Outside the Mail)*	(1)	Free or Nominal Rate Outside-County Copies included on PS Form 3541	16	7
	(2)	Free or Nominal Rate In-County Copies Included on PS Form 3541	0	0
	(3)	Free or Nominal Rate Copies Mailed at Other Classes Through the USPS (e.g. First-Class Mail)	0	0
	(4)	Free or Nominal Rate Distribution Outside the Mail *(Carriers or other means)*	0	0
e. Total Free or Nominal Rate Distribution *(Sum of 15d (1), (2), (3) and (4))*		▶	16	7
f. Total Distribution *(Sum of 15c and 15e)*		▶	72	50
g. Copies not Distributed *(See Instructions to Publishers #4 (page #3))*		▶	16	17
h. Total *(Sum of 15f and g)*		▶	88	67
i. Percent Paid *(15c divided by 15f times 100)*		▶	77.77%	86%

* If you are claiming electronic copies, go to line 16 on page 3. If you are not claiming electronic copies, skip to line 17 on page 3.

16. Electronic Copy Circulation

	Average No. Copies Each Issue During Preceding 12 Months	No. Copies of Single Issue Published Nearest to Filing Date
a. Paid Electronic Copies ▶		
b. Total Paid Print Copies (Line 15c) + Paid Electronic Copies (Line 16a) ▶		
c. Total Print Distribution (Line 15f) + Paid Electronic Copies (Line 16a) ▶		
d. Percent Paid (Both Print & Electronic Copies) (16b divided by 16c × 100) ▶		

☒ I certify that 50% of all my distributed copies (electronic and print) are paid above a nominal price.

17. Publication of Statement of Ownership

☒ If the publication is a general publication, publication of this statement is required. Will be printed in the DECEMBER 2021 issue of this publication.   ☐ Publication not required.

18. Signature and Title of Editor, Publisher, Business Manager, or Owner

Malathi Samayan   Malathi Samayan - Distribution Controller

Date: 9/18/2021

I certify that all information furnished on this form is true and complete. I understand that anyone who furnishes false or misleading information on this form or who omits material or information requested on the form may be subject to criminal sanctions (including fines and imprisonment) and/or civil sanctions (including civil penalties).

PS Form **3526**, July 2014 (Page 3 of 4)   PRIVACY NOTICE: See our privacy policy on www.usps.com

9780323809245